Seydou Coulibaly

Angioscan diagnosis

Seydou Coulibaly

Angioscan diagnosis

of a peripheral superficial arteriovenous malformation of the elbow in a newborn at Mali Hospital

ScienciaScripts

Imprint

Cover image: www.ingimage.com

This book is a translation from the original published under ISBN 978-620-6-70075-3.

Publisher:
Sciencia Scripts
is a trademark of
Dodo Books Indian Ocean Ltd. and OmniScriptum S.R.L publishing group

120 High Road, East Finchley, London, N2 9ED, United Kingdom
Str. Armeneasca 28/1, office 1, Chisinau MD-2012, Republic of Moldova, Europe
Printed at: see last page
ISBN: 978-620-8-02410-9

Contents

DEDICATION 2
ACKNOWLEDGEMENTS 3
TRIBUTES TO THE MEMBERS OF THE JURY 4
INTRODUCTION 6
CHAPTER 1 8
CHAPTER 2 43
CHAPTER 3 54
CHAPTER 4 60
REFERENCES 61
Summary 64

DEDICATION

I dedicate this work :

To my father, the late Oumar COULIBALY, I am very proud to be counted among your sons, you fought so that I could go to school and you instilled in us the rules of good conduct, dignity, respect for human beings and wisdom. I would have liked everything to have happened in your presence, but God decided otherwise. Rest in peace, dear Dad.

To my mother Kadidia COULIBALY, Courageous and devoted. You surrounded us with attention and affection that always brought us comfort and consolation. You never stopped caring about our future. Words fail me today to express all my gratitude for your sacrifices and the hard work you endured to bring us up. I can never thank you enough. This work is the fruit of your efforts. Only God can reward you. May God, the Almighty, grant you long life, good health and above all happiness. May he give us the means to fight for you in life.

To my wife Sira KEÏTA, my sons Seydina oumar, Hassane and Housseyni; this work is yours. You have been patient throughout this study in the hope that one day you will be rewarded. May Allah bless you and your family.

To my brothers, sisters and cousins, whom I won't mention here for fear of leaving someone out. Family unity is priceless, and may it remain the primary objective for all of us. For all your support and as a token of your love, I dedicate this work to you.

To my brothers and all the HAÏDARA family in Bla, Bamako, Ouagadougou and Abidjan, thank you for your presence, your patience and your support. I will never regret the education I received in the family. Please accept here all my affection and gratitude.

To my aunts, Nana YATOURA, Hawa DIALLO, Aminata TRAORE and Fatoumata TRAORE, it is thanks to you that I am where I am today. I have never lacked support and affection in the family. Words will never be enough to express what you mean to me. I can only humbly say thank you. May GOD bless you and keep you with us for as long as possible so that we can show you all our gratitude.

To my brother, Mr Mamadou HAÏDARA, thank you for the esteem and respect you have shown me. The good GOD will be grateful for your innumerable services to your fellow men.

ACKNOWLEDGEMENTS

I thank ALLAH, the almighty, the most merciful, who has given me the chance to live this moment, the strength and the will to do this work. For so much love, so much grace and your mercy towards me, a poor sinner.

To our master, Professor CAMARA Mody Abdoulaye, your knowledge of medicine and medical imaging in particular, and your ability to pass on knowledge have set an example for me, and it is an honour to train alongside you. Please find here the expression of my deep respect and my sincere thanks.

To Pr TRAORE Mohamed Maba, Dr Sounkalo TRAORE, Dr DIARRA Hawa, Dr TOURE Boubacar, Dr MAIGA Oumou, Dr KONATE Zakaria, Dr KOUYATE Mamadou Mary; thank you for your availability, your valuable advice and the quality of the teaching you provided.

To all the secretaries, technicians, interns and DES in the medical imaging department at Mali Hospital, CSRef CV and CSRef CVI.

To my friends and graduates: Dr GACKOU Mahamadou, Dr KEITA Siaka, Dr Bakary D. COULIBALY, Boubacar TRAORE, Dr Boubacar SYLLA, Dr TRAORE Adama, Dr KAMIA Boureima, Dr DOUMBIA Modibo, Dr SANOGO Modibo, Dr FADIGA Sory Ibrahim, Dr CAMARA Nagnoumagué and Dr FOMBA Moussa.

To the entire $9^{\text{ième}}$ class of the numérus clausus named Promotion Feu Pr. Ibrahima ALWATA.

To all the members of the association of pupils, health students and sympathisers of the cercle de BLA and the association of pupils and students of the commune of NIALA and sympathisers.

To our masters and guides, and to all the teachers of the FMOS. I am the product of your investment. Please accept my gratitude.

To all those who have helped me in one way or another.

To all those I may have forgotten: I wish you all the best with no hard feelings.

You have supported me in one way or another, and I can only sum it all up in one word: thank you, may Allah reward you.

TRIBUTES TO THE MEMBERS OF THE JURY

To our Master and Chairman of the jury :

Professor Adama Diaman KEITA

[1]¼ Professor of Radiology and Medical Imaging
[1]¼ Specialist in forensic and parasitic imaging,
[1]¼ Head of the radiology and medical imaging department at the CHU du Point-G,
[1]¼ Former Head of DER Medicine and Medical Specialties at FMOS
[1]¼ Former Rector of the University of Science, Techniques and Technology of Bamako (USTTB).

Honourable Counsel

We are very honoured by the spontaneity with which you agreed to chair this jury, despite your busy schedule.

Your scientific rigour, your high-quality teaching and your simplicity have made you a great master admired by all.

Please accept, dear Master, the expression of our great respect and our sincere thanks.

May the Lord grant you health and longevity.

[1]¼ Full Professor of Thoracic and Cardiovascular Surgery (CTCV) at FMOS,
[1]¼ Hospital practitioner at Mali Hospital
[1]¼ Member of the Surgical Society of Mali (SOCHIMA)
[1]¼ Founding member of the Society of Thoracic and Cardiovascular Surgery.

Dear Master,

We're lucky to have you on the jury, despite your busy schedule.

We were impressed by your humanism, your availability and your simplicity.

Please find here dear master the expression of our sincere thanks[1] ¼ Head of Paediatrics at Mali Hospital.

[1]¼ Diploma in neonatology and neonatal resuscitation
[1]¼ Degree in nutrition from Boston University
[1]¼ Diploma in pneumology and paediatric allergology
[1]¼ Master of research in paediatrics,
[1]¼ Member of the French Paediatric and Allergology Society

Dear Master,

We would like to thank you for the spontaneity with which you agreed to sit on this dissertation jury,

We always admired your scientific and social qualities,

Please accept our sincere thanks and gratitude.

To our Master and Co-director :
Dr Abdoulaye KONE

[1]¼ Assistant Professor at the FMOS
[1]¼ Radiologist and hospital practitioner at the Pasteur polyclinic in Bamako
[1]¼ Inter-university diploma (DIU) in whole-body magnetic resonance imaging at the University of Paris Descartes, Paris V
[1]¼ Diplôme de formation Médicale spécialisée Approfondie (DFMSA) at the Université Pierre et Marie Curie, Paris VI.
[1]¼ Member of learned societies: SOMIM, SFR and SRANF

Dear Master,
Passing on knowledge to others is an act of faith.
In you, we have found the love of a job well done and a strong sense of duty.
This work is the fruit of your perfect commitment and expertise.
Your highly valued social character makes you a person of exceptional class.
You can count on our availability and our deep gratitude.

To our Master and Director :
Professor Mody Abdoulaye CAMARA

[1]¼ Radiologist and hospital practitioner at Mali Hospital,
[1]¼ Lecturer in Radiology and Medical Imaging at FMOS,[1] ¼ Head of the Medical Imaging Department at Mali Hospital.
[1]¼ Diplôme de formation Médicale spécialisée Approfondie (DFMSA).
[1]¼ Member of learned societies: SOMIM, SFR and SRANF

Dear Master,
Passing on knowledge to others is an act of faith.
In you, we have found the love of a job well done and a strong sense of duty.
This work is the fruit of your perfect commitment and expertise.
Your highly appreciated social nature makes you an exceptional character. You can count on our availability and our deep gratitude.

INTRODUCTION

Arteriovenous malformations are defined by the existence of congenital arteriovenous shunts. The imbalance between arterial inflow and outflow leads to dilatation, sometimes aneurysmal, of the venous drainage sector, but also within the nidus and afferent arteries [1].

AVMs are most commonly seen in the paediatric population. They consist of a direct shunt known as a true fistula. The flow rate is very high and major venous dilatation is in the foreground 1[er] . These are rare lesions with a high haemorrhagic potential [1].

The prevalence of all forms of vascular malformations is estimated at 1.5% in the general population [2]. They account for approximately 7% of benign lesions. The majority develop in the brain and cervical region [3]. Peripheral lesions (extracerebral and extra-spinal) are rare, accounting for 5-10% [2], particularly in the upper limbs [4].

Arteriovenous malformations (AVMs) may be asymptomatic, but they never regress spontaneously. These arteriovenous malformations are associated with the highest rate of complications [2].

Improved access to magnetic resonance imaging (MRI) has led to a significant increase in the number of AVMs diagnosed in recent years [5]. However, arteriography used to be the gold standard. However, advances in magnetic resonance angiography (MRA) sequences, particularly in dynamic acquisition, mean that it is now the gold standard for confirming the type of malformation and monitoring patients' progress [6].

In children, echodoppler is the first-line examination used to confirm the diagnosis. It also plays a role in sclerotherapy, but MRI is the examination of choice [7]. Angioscanner still has a limited role to play, but technical advances may lead to this modality playing an increasing role in the near future [8].

The various treatment options for AVMs need to be carefully evaluated on the basis of numerous criteria specific to the malformation and the patient. Treatment options include simple observation, endovascular embolisation, surgical resection and radiosurgical irradiation [9]. Localisation in the upper limbs poses a therapeutic problem [8].

Using a case report and a review of the literature, we will discuss the diagnostic and therapeutic aspects of angioscanning raised by this entity.

Objectives

General objective :

To determine the contribution of angio-CT in the diagnosis of arteriovenous malformation in newborns.

Specific objectives :

- ✓ Describe the CT aspects of superficial arteriovenous malformation.
- ✓ A review of the literature on superficial arteriovenous malformations.

CHAPTER 1

1. GENERAL

1.1.History

The history of superficial vascular anomalies is a long terminological saga in which the term "angiomas" has long prevailed to designate this succession of benign diseases, although this does not rule out their possible seriousness. These congenital or acquired anomalies are clinically heterogeneous, with long-standing group specificities [10].

From antiquity to the 18th century, there was no mention of angiomas. Similar words were used in all languages, such as envy, voglia, estigma, birthmark, all of which stigmatised mothers who, during their pregnancy, had unhealthy thoughts, veritable teratogenic thoughts capable of marking their child with spots or deformities! [10].

In the XIXe century, superficial vascular lesions were referred to as nvus maternus (always the idea of involving those unfortunate mothers!), nvus sanguineus, nvus vascularis, nvus venous. **Virchow** seems to be the creator of the term "angioma", but he failed in his attempt to classify them, even though he had clearly distinguished lesions due to cell proliferation from others resulting from vascular dilatation [10].

At the beginning of the XXe century, the idea of differentiating between vascular tumours and vascular malformations was gaining ground. **Malan** devoted his life to what he called "angiodysplasias". **Weiss and Enzinger** favoured the term haemangioma, but used it to refer to benign tumours as well as malignant lesions or vascular malformations [10].

Exploration techniques are developing and multiple classifications are appearing, with clinical, histological, haemodynamic, angio-graphic, embryological and biological bases. However, there is still a great deal of confusion [10].

In 1982, Mulliken and Glowacki proposed their "biological" classification, the basis of the modern classification, essentially based on cell kinetic data. It distinguishes between haemangiomas (vascular tumours that develop through cell proliferation) and vascular malformations (composed of altered and dilated vessels, but whose parietal cells are not proliferating) [10].

The term "angioma" can no longer represent all the superficial vascular anomalies it used to cover, because the suffix "ome" implies the notion of cellular hyperplasia, of tumour: in this classification, only haemangioma is an angioma [10].

The term lymphangioma is also inappropriate, as it refers to a lymphatic malformation anomaly, whether the lesion is microcystic or macrocystic.

The first two **International Workshops on Vascular Anomalies** were held in 1976 and 1978. Initially, three countries took part (United States: Professor John Mulliken, a craniofacial surgeon; United Kingdom: Professor Anthony Young, a vascular surgeon; and France: Professor Jean-Jacques Merland, a pioneer in interventional neuroradiology). The beginnings were informal. However, the arrival of new specialists - doctors, surgeons, radiologists and biologists - soon enabled different approaches and information to be compared [10].

This is encouraging the emergence of multidisciplinary groups in various countries.

Terminology discussions are at the forefront (we need to find a simple common language). Ongoing workshops, held every two years (even-numbered years), enable data to be reconciled and collated [10].

Finally, the current binary classification into vascular tumours and vascular malformations, derived from that of Mulliken and Glowacki (Figure 13), was adopted at the Rome workshop in 1996 [2,3].

Clinical and histological knowledge is improving. So are haemodynamic and radiological data [7].

Biological advances are deciphering the mechanisms of haemangiogenesis; angiogenic factors and regulatory cytokines involved in tumours and malformations are being analysed. Molecular biology is deciphering the gene mutations involved in certain familial forms of vascular malformations [7-10].

The International Society for the Study of Vascular Anomalies (ISSVA) was founded in 1992 as an extension of the workshop, which continues every two years. In 2008, the 17^{e} workshop was held in Boston with multidisciplinary participation from five continents. The 18^{e} workshop was held in Brussels in 2010 [2].

1.2.Classification: [11]

Until the early 1970s, the term "angioma" was used to describe a wide variety of unrelated superficial vascular anomalies for which treatment was either non-existent or often inappropriate. In 1976, the work of Merland's team at Lariboisière and Mulliken's team in Boston led to a logical and simple classification based on clinical, histological and haemodynamic criteria [11].

This classification divided "angiomas" into two main groups:

- haemangiomas of newborns and infants, which are immature haemangiomas,
- and superficial vascular malformations proper which are mature malformations which, unlike haemangiomas, will never regress but will progress throughout life more or less rapidly depending on their histological nature and haemodynamics [11].

However, some haemangiomas do not have the usual clinical course, and histology and biology have enabled new entities to be identified [11].

There are always two groups:

- On the one hand, vascular tumours
- And superficial vascular malformations [11].

Vascular tumours are mainly represented by infantile haemangiomas, which are the most common, but there are also other vascular tumours such as congenital haemangiomas, tufted angiomas and kaposiform haemangioendotheliomas (Figure 4) [11].

Vascular malformations may involve the capillaries, which give rise to planar angiomas, the veins, which give rise to venous malformations formerly known as venous angiomas, or the lymphatics, which are responsible for lymphatic malformations classically known as lymphangiomas, which are most often cystic [11].

Vascular malformations can develop at the expense of arteries, giving rise to the dreaded arteriovenous malformations (AVMs) [11].

Capillary, venous and lymphatic malformations are haemodynamically inactive, whereas AVMs are haemodynamically active with a severe potential for progression [11].

Each of these malformations has its own specific clinical picture, requiring specific investigations and appropriate treatment [11].

There are complex vascular malformations which may combine capillary, venous, lymphatic and arterial damage in varying ways, posing difficult management problems [11].

In the majority of cases, clinical diagnosis is essential, and the diagnosis and type of malformation can be confirmed by questioning, history of the malformation and clinical examination [11].

At each consultation, a photograph is taken and filed in the patient's file. Specialised examinations such as echodoppler, CT scan, magnetic resonance imaging (MRI), arteriography and MRI angiography are sometimes required to confirm the diagnosis and help with treatment [11]. Each type of anomaly has its own diagnostic and therapeutic approach [11].

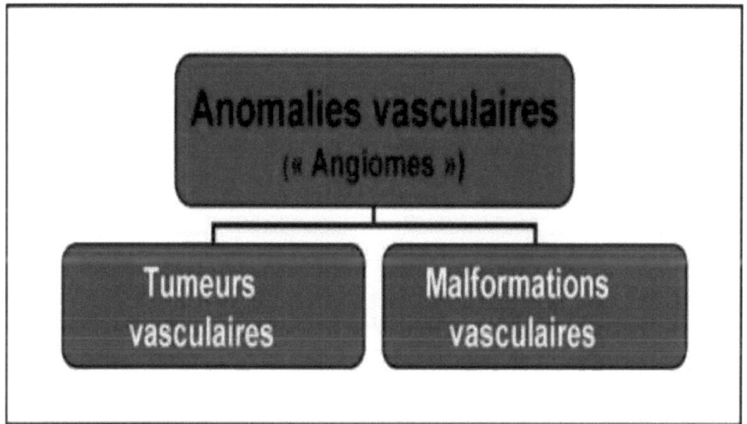

Figure 1: Classification of superficial vascular anomalies [15].

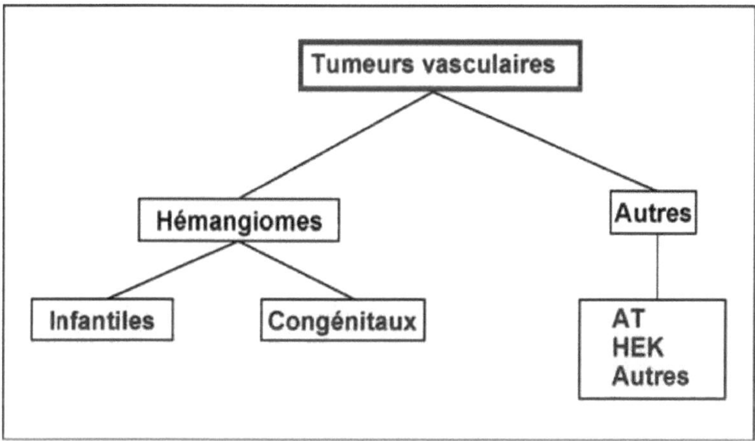

Figure 2: Classification of vascular tumours [12].

AT: tufted angioma; HEK: kaposiform haemangioendothelioma

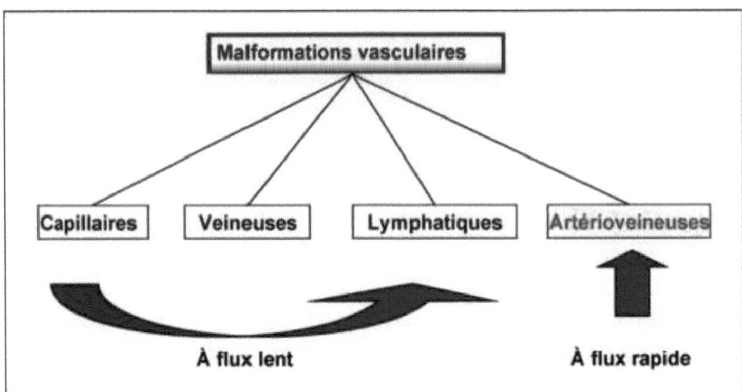

Figure 3: Classification of vascular malformations [12].

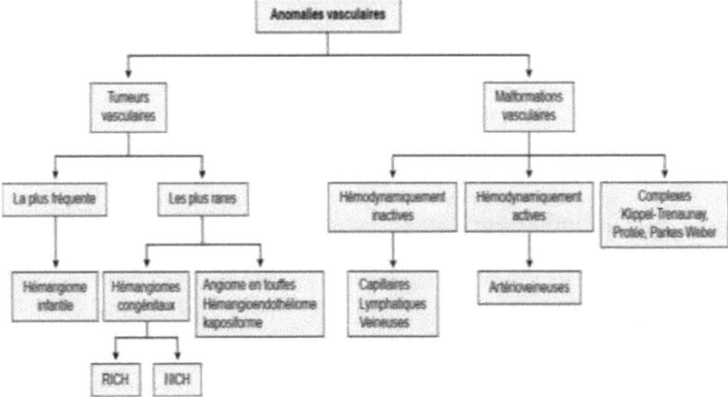

Figure 4: Classification of vascular anomalies. RICH: rapidly involuting congenital haemangioma; NICH: non involuting congenital haemangioma [11].

A new classification was therefore carried out by the International Society for the Study of Vascular Anomalies (ISSVA) in 2014, revised in 2018 [12].

Table 1: Classification of vascular anomalies according to the 20th workshop of the ISSVA [12].

Vascular anomalies				
Tumours	**Vascular malformation**			
Benign Locally aggressive or borderline Malignant	**Simple**	**Combined**	**Large vessels**	**Associated with other anomalies**
	Capillary malformation Lymphatic malformation Venous	MCV, MCL MLV,		

	malformation Arteriovenous malformation Arteriovenous fistula	MCLV MCAV MCLAV Other		

Table 2: Classification of arteriovenous malformations according to the 20th ISSVA workshop [12].

Simple vascular malformations
Arteriovenous malformations (AVMs)
Sporadic
MAP2K1
In HHT
(HHT1 ENG, HHT2 ACVRL1, HHT3, JPHT SMAD4)
In MC-AVM
RASA1 / EPHB4
Other
Arteriovenous fistulas (congenital)
Sporadic
MAP2K1
In HHT
(HHT1 ENG, HHT2 ACVRL1, HHT3, JPHT SMAD4)
In CM-AVM
RASA1 / EPHB4
Other

1.3.Epidemiology

The incidence in the United States is 1.34 per 100,000 person-years. Although the true prevalence rate is higher due to the clinically silent disease, as it is estimated that only 12% become symptomatic. The mortality rate is 10-15% of patients who experience a haemorrhage [1].

Morbidity varies from around 30-50%. There is no sexual predilection. Despite its congenital origin, the clinical presentation occurs most often in young adults [1].

1.4.Anatomical reminder :

❖ **Arteries of the upper limb**:

The right subclavian artery arises behind the sternoclavicular joint, from the bifurcation of the brachiocephalic arterial trunk into this axis and into the right primitive carotid artery. On the left, the subclavian artery arises directly from the superior surface of the aortic arch. This artery describes a curve with an inferior concavity on the pleural dome, crosses the interscalene defilement and then insinuates itself between the clavicle and the external edge of the first rib,

downstream of which it becomes the axillary artery, as far as the inferior edge of the pectoralis major where the brachial artery then begins. The brachial artery runs along the anterior aspect of the upper arm and elbow to the level of the bicipital tuberosity of the radius, where it bifurcates into the radial artery and the ulnar artery. The radial artery, a branch of the external division of the brachial artery, arises classically 3 cm below the elbow joint and runs along the radius, in the anterior compartment of the forearm, as far as the pulse groove; it crosses the radiocarpal space and reaches, on the dorsal surface of the carpus, the upper end of the 1st interosseous space, where it anastomoses, in the palm of the hand, with the ulnopalmar artery, a branch of the ulnar artery, to form the deep palmar arch. The ulnar artery, an internal bifurcation branch of the brachial artery, runs in the medial part of the anterior compartment of the forearm, from the elbow crease to the palm of the hand, where it anastomoses with the radiopalmar artery, a branch of the radial artery, to form the superficial palmar arch [13].
The deep palmar arch describes a wide loop which projects opposite the heads of the metacarpals; in particular, it gives rise to four palmar interosseous arteries which anastomose with the digital arteries at the commissure of the fingers. The superficial palmar arch describes an angular loop with inferior convexity, projecting from the carpus and the heads of the 3rd and 4th metacarpals; it gives rise to the digital arteries destined for the last four fingers. Dorsal collaterals, mainly from the radial (more rarely from the ulnar), form the dorsal arch of the carpus (Figure 5A) [13].

❖ **Anatomical variations**

Variations in arterial vascularisation of the upper limbs are relatively rare, but nevertheless more frequent than in the lower limbs. They are represented in particular by an early division, above the condylar space, of the brachial artery (high birth of the radial artery - in 10% of individuals -, high birth of the ulnar artery or premature birth of these two axes). The right subclavian artery, which arises directly from the aorta after the left subclavian artery (arteria lusoria), may have a retro-oesophageal course. Duplication of the brachial artery is another rare occurrence. On the other hand, the possibilities of supplementation, via anastomoses and perforators, between the different arches of the hand are subject to fairly frequent anatomical variations [1,2].

❖ **Veins of the upper limb :**

o **Deep veins :**

The deep veins of the upper limb are satellites of the arteries, and there are two per artery. Only the axillary artery is accompanied by a single venous trunk: the axillary vein (Figure 5B) [13].

o **Superficial veins**

There are three superficial veins in the forearm. The median radial vein is the most commonly used for the creation of arteriovenous fistulas. It divides at the elbow into the medial cephalic root and the lateral basilic root. Medial to this is the superficial ulnar vein. The external or accessory radial vein is the most external. The external radial vein, the bifurcated median radial vein and the superficial ulnar vein form the venous "M" at the elbow. In the upper arm, two veins therefore arise directly from the venous "M", one internal, the basilic vein, the proximal portion of which becomes deep, and the other external, the cephalic vein.

The union of the deep humeral veins and the basilic vein forms the axillary vein, while the cephalic vein drains into the subclavian vein after describing a final arch (Figure 5B) [13].

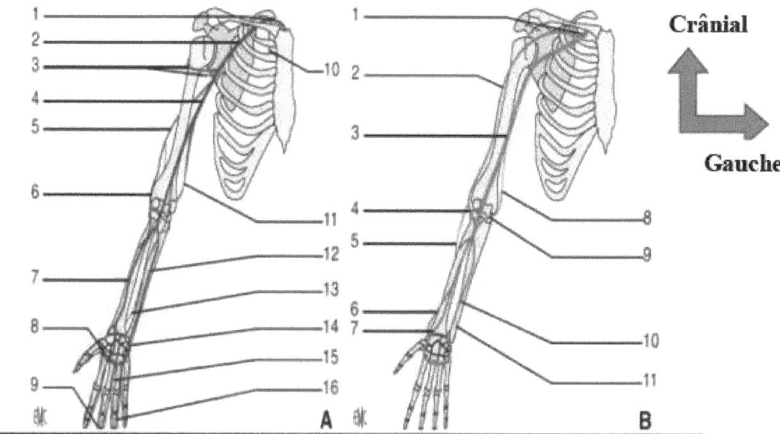

Figure 5: Diagram showing the simplified anatomy of the arteries (A), deep veins and superficial veins (B) of the upper limb [13].

A. 1. Subclavian artery; 2. Axillary artery; 3. Circumflex artery; 4. Brachial artery; 5. Deep brachial artery; 6. Radial collateral artery; 7. Radial artery; 8. superficial palmar arch; 9. radial palmar digital artery; 10. internal thoracic artery; 11. ulnar collateral artery; 12. ulnar artery; 13. anterior interosseous artery; 14. deep palmar arch; 15. common digital artery; 16. ulnar palmar digital artery.

B. 1. Subclavian vein; 2. cephalic vein; 3. brachial veins (x2); 4. medial cephalic vein; 5. accessory radial vein; 6. superficial radial vein; 7. radial veins (x2); 8. basilic vein; 9. medial basilic vein; 10. ulnar veins (x2); 11. superficial ulnar vein.

1.5.Means of exploration :

Diagnosis is based on clinical and ultrasound data.

Other complementary examinations, in particular cross-sectional imaging (MRI and/or CT), are necessary to confirm the diagnosis and determine the locoregional extension of the AVM [14].

1.5.1. Doppler ultrasound

Doppler ultrasound is the first-line complementary examination. It confirms a poorly defined, non-tissue lesion with rapid flow, arterialisation of venous flows, very high velocities, high diastolic flow, low resistance index <0.5, useful for distinguishing flat angiomas or other vascular malformations (lymphatic or venous, which have slower flow) from quiescent AVMs. Comparative flow confirms arterial hyperflow. Measurement of this upstream arterial flow allows the evolution of the malformation to be monitored, but is very operator-dependent [14].

1.5.2. Angio-MRI and Angioscan :

MRI can be used to assess the depth of invasion of the AVM, and arterial angioscanner provides a good analysis of the angioarchitecture and any tissue and bone invasion [14].

Pre- or post-treatment monitoring is carried out using these non-invasive tests, which are of course combined with clinical examinations [14].

MRI is preferred in children because it is non-irradiating. It generally requires sedation in children under 6 years of age [14].

1.5.3. X-ray :

Standard radiography of the affected limb is useful for looking for intraosseous localisations, in cases of clinical suspicion [14].

If there is inequality in the length of the lower limbs, radiomography of the limbs should be requested in order to establish this [14].

1.5.4. Angiography

Angiography is not recommended as a first-line treatment. It should be decided in a specialist multidisciplinary consultation, as in some cases it may be useful in deciding on treatment. The aim is to determine the angioarchitecture of the lesion [14].

1.5.5. Histopathological examination and molecular analysis

Biopsy is generally contraindicated in AVMs. It can be complicated by heavy bleeding and can trigger a progressive relapse. It may be discussed and carried out by a specialist multidisciplinary team for the purposes of :

- **Histopathological analysis**: this will highlight arteriovenous shunts and the absence of tumour proliferation, in the event of diagnostic doubt (with a malignant tumour in particular) [14] ;
- **Molecular analysis:** search for somatic mutations in the *KRAS, NRAS, BRAF* and *MAP2K1* genes. At present, this analysis is on the borderline between research and care, with targeted therapies under study [14].

1.6.Different types of vascular malformation :

These are anomalies of morphogenesis, all congenital and present at birth. They grow with age and never regress [15].

Clinical features such as warmth of the skin around the malformation, palpation of a thrill, and hearing of a murmur should be sought out and reported: they point to an arteriovenous malformation. The emptying of the malformation when the affected limb is raised is in favour of a purely venous malformation, as is the swelling of a lesion in the face when the head is bent downwards or when a limb is placed in the downward position. The presence of capillary malformation, superficial venous dilatations, asymmetry of limb length and/or circumference should be noted. In the case of AVMs, look for signs of heart failure [2].

Two main groups can be distinguished on the basis of haemodynamic criteria:

1.6.1. Slow-flow vascular malformations

a. Capillary malformations :

There are two types, telangiectasias and flat angiomas, and they are thought to be the most common superficial vascular malformations [2].

a.1. Flat angioma or "wine stain

A planar angioma is a spot of variable colour ranging from pale pink to dark purple, macular, with fairly well-defined contours, present at birth and never fading spontaneously. With age, its texture may change and it becomes a palpable, thick, grainy scarlet sheet [16].

This is the most common capillary malformation and manifests itself as an intense red lesion on the skin in the neonatal period, which is cold and not beating [2].

It will gradually fade without regressing, with the exception of the mid-frontal "angel's kiss" and cervical "stork bite" forms, which disappear in one to two years [2].

In neonates, it is sometimes difficult to distinguish between a PA and an incipient haemangioma. It is important to be wary of false, warm, flat angiomas, which are in fact the skin covering of an arteriovenous malformation [2].

Some angiomas change in adults. They thicken, become vinous and are surmounted by purplish nodules. They have no regional or general repercussions and only cause cosmetic damage [2].

a.2. Syndromes associated with angioma plana :

PA may reflect a more complex syndrome:

❖ **Sturge Weber Krabbe (SWK) syndrome**: In the face, involvement of the territory of the first branch of the trigeminal nerve, especially if there is associated involvement of the upper eyelid, should raise fears of association with angioma of the magpie mother and glaucoma. Cerebro-meningeal involvement is responsible for epilepsy, which is often early and severe, with psychomotor retardation. Involvement of the second or third branch of the trigeminal nerve is not associated with such complications [16].

❖ **Klippel Trenaunay syndrome:** Certain flat angiomas of the limbs are accompanied by a progressive increase in the volume and length of the limb and varicose veins. The prognosis of this complex capillaroveinous malformation is often serious in terms of aesthetics and function [16].

❖ **Cobb's syndrome:** This combines a cutaneous AVM, often in the form of a planar pseudoangioma, with a spinal cord AVM and sometimes a vertebral or paraspinal intramuscular AVM in the same metamerium [2].

Neurological complications may begin in childhood. MRI, MRI angiography and arteriography are used to assess the condition. Treatment depends on the location of the spinal cord angioma: embolisation or surgical excision **[17]**.

❖ **Proteus syndrome:** This syndrome presents a particular picture with angioma planus, congenital hypertrophy of a limb linked to lymphoedema or soft tissue hypertrophy and sometimes other anomalies **[17]**.

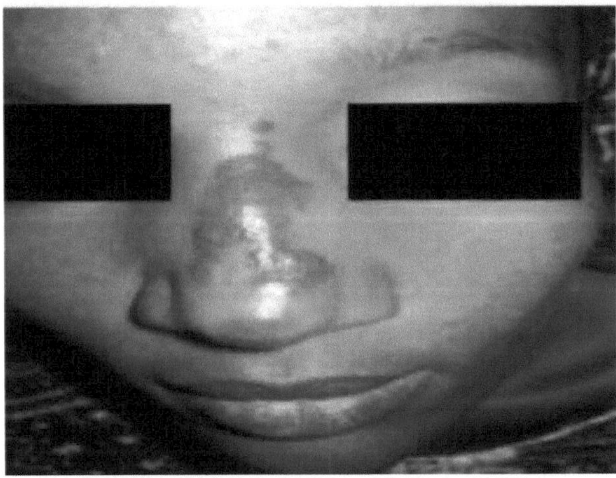

Figure 6: plane angioma of the nose [8].

Histology :

In children, capillary malformation manifests itself as a simple dilation of superficial dermal capillaries. These capillaries are normal structures and appear to be normal in number [16].

In adults, as the lesion thickens, the wall of the capillaries becomes fibrous, resembling a venule. They are found throughout the dermis and sometimes the hypodermis. The apparent number of vascular sections visible on a cross-

sectional plane and their diameter are clearly increased [16].
Sometimes, the vessels are packed together to create a "cavernous" appearance with dividing walls. Hypertrophic capillary malformations combine capillary dilatations in the dermis with venous bundles in the deep dermis and hypodermis. The prominent nodules that may appear on capillary malformations are made up of bundles of large-diameter vessels with a fibrous wall, sometimes simulating a localised dermal arteriovenous malformation [2].

a.3. Telangiectasias

These are always dermal capillary dysplasias but with a particular morphology: linear or stellate telangiectasia "stellate angioma". Some small linear capillary angiomas are surmounted by a hyperkeratotic epidermis, rough to the touch and which does not fade on in vitro pressure: angiokeratomas [2].
These isolated capillary hyperplasias are distinguished from the capillary angiomatosis known as Rendu-Osler disease (hereditary haemorrhagic telangiectasia) [2].

b. Venous malformations

Venous malformations (MV) give the skin or mucous membranes a bluish appearance. They are soft and cold to the touch. Venous pouches swell when the patient is in the upright position or during exercise, and are easily emptied during compression manoeuvres. The latter is an excellent distinctive sign. These malformations are painful when tension is applied [18].
VD involves all planes (cutaneous, subcutaneous, mucosal or submucosal tissues, muscles, synovium and bone). Visible" surface extension is not correlated with deep extension [18].
Their topography is ubiquitous, with a predilection for the cervico-cephalic or temporo-masseterial regions (Figure 7). Approximately 20% of large facial malformations are associated with intracranial venous anomalies that develop asymptomatically [18].
Hepatic haemangiomas, vertebral haemangiomas, aneurysmal bone cysts and cerebral cavernomas belong to the family of venous malformations.
Cerebral cavernomas are true pathological venous angiomas, whereas "venous angiomas", a misnomer, are asymptomatic cerebral venous anomalies. Vertebral angiomas are venous and fatty in asymptomatic forms and capillary-venous in aggressive forms [2].

b.1. Histology

They are made up of abnormal veins, some of whose walls are devoid of "alpha-actin positive" smooth muscle cells. They form a complex network of thin-walled venous cavities [2].

b.2. Clinical presentation and complications :

VD does not present a progressive flare-up as such, but increases progressively from birth to adulthood, as if its constituent elements were developing one after the other [2].

Characteristic thrombosis episodes are responsible for painful attacks lasting a fortnight, progressing to a fibrous and calcified transformation [2].

Phleboliths are the stigmata. The thrombotic process is the consequence of localised intravascular consumption (LIC) within the malformation [2].

In contrast to Kasabach-Merritt syndrome, this process relatively spares platelets. It is due to a defect in the release of the endothelial activator of fibrinolysis, combining an increase in fibrin degradation products with a drop in fibrinogen [2].

Spontaneous haematomas are rarer and secondary to coagulation disorders. The LIC phenomenon may be complicated by disseminated intravascular consumption (DIC) leading to massive haemorrhage. Bleeding occurs after the malformation has been attacked by injury, a change in hormonal profile (pregnancy, contraceptive use) or inappropriate surgery [2].

Venous distension progresses throughout life and is responsible for aesthetic, functional and psychological damage [2].

Extension of the temporomasseterine form to the floor of the mouth can lead to orthodontic problems. Involvement of the orbit (via the inferior orbital fissure) and the pharyngolaryngeal space is accompanied respectively by exophthalmos on exertion (due to swelling of the extra-conical intra-orbital venous pockets) and dyspnoea [2].

Located in the aero-digestive tract, VD is responsible for sleep apnoea.

The orbito-palpebral form causes exophthalmos on exertion, which eventually leads to amblyopia [2].

Large, disabling lingual VD leads to dis-occlusion.

VD of the limbs and trunk is generally well tolerated in childhood. However, as they progress, they are accompanied by a series of functional signs that interfere with normal movements. They sometimes affect an entire limb segment and take on considerable proportions.

Located in the lower limbs, secondary amyotrophy and an equinus attitude are a handicap when walking. They are often mistakenly confused with Klippel-Trenaunay syndrome [2].

Knee VD is responsible for recurrent haemarthrosis in cases of intra-articular extension, leading to functional impotence.

Located on the finger, the bluish, cold pockets are sometimes difficult to empty with manual compression. Phleboliths deform the fingers and even the palm.

They cause considerable functional damage [2].
Vulvar VD is rare but symptomatic, with dyspareunia and dysmenorrhoea. It increases in size during menstruation or pregnancy as a result of mechanical venous hyperpressure and increased pelvic blood volume. Painful thrombosis accompanies its development [2].
Close to the nipple, the malformation impedes the development of the lactation organ [2].

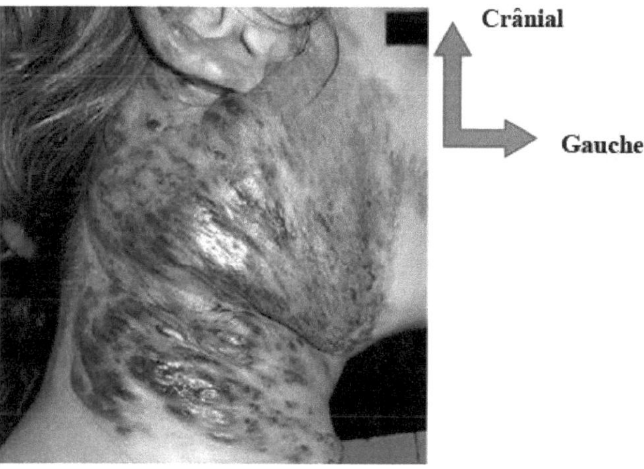

Figure 7: Cervico-facial venous malformation. Superficial venous pockets are blue and swell with slope [2].

b.3 Imaging

Ultrasound :

It shows liquid lakes sometimes associated with dilated and sinuous peripheral venous structures. These lakes present very slow flows which are often imperceptible even with very sensitive Doppler settings. The search for fluid movements is facilitated by compression movements undermined by the ultrasound probe, allowing the Iogettes to be seen emptying and filling with fluid. In B mode, the discovery of a phlebolith (image of compact calcification within the malformation) is very typical [21].

MRI :

The generally infiltrative nature of venous malformations suggests that MRI should be performed to assess deep extension (intramuscular, intra-articular, intra-perineal, etc.) and relationships with neighbouring organs [21].
This assessment is essential if surgical treatment is planned. Images should be acquired in at least two spatial planes (axial/coronal or axial/sagittal) in T2

weighting with suppression of the fat signal: the venous malformation, because of its highly hydrated nature, can be clearly distinguished from adjacent structures [19-20]. This is the best test for showing sheets and pockets with hypersignal on T2-weighted sequences [21].

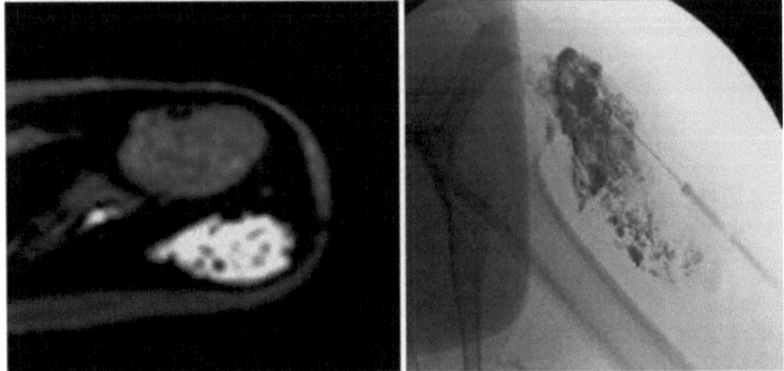

Figure 8: T2 MRI: venous malformation in the left shoulder before and after sclerosis [19].

c. Cystic lymphatic malformations

These are hemodynamically inactive congenital malformations, consisting of abnormal lymphatic vessels and cysts of variable morphology. They generally appear in early childhood but are sometimes diagnosed antenatally by ultrasound [20]. They are classically divided into lymphatic malformations :

- Microcystic (tissue form), made up of cysts smaller than 2 cm^3
- Macrocystic (cystic form) formed by cysts larger than 2 cm^3 - And mixed [20].

The cystic form appears as a hard, renitent, well-limited swelling, located preferentially in the cervico-encephalic and axillary regions (Figure 9). The macrocysts are often multiple and communicating. The skin is normal, with no increase in heat [20].

The tissue form appears as a poorly defined infiltrating patch of skin or mucous membrane, covered with translucent or blackish vesicles. It occurs preferentially on the face or proximal limbs [20].

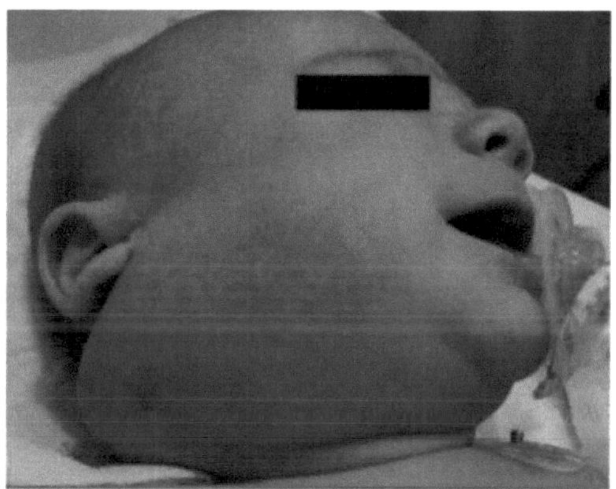

Figure 9: Cervicofacial macrocystic lymphatic malformations [22].

c.1. Histology :

Cystic and tissue MLK derive from the same origin. During embryogenesis, an anomaly in the formation of the lymphatic sacs gives rise to the cystic form, predominantly in the cervical region. An anomaly in the development of the primitive lymphatic vessels gives rise to the tissue form. The proliproliferation of lymphatic vessels is due to several factors. Increased secretion of VEGF-C (vascular endothelial growth factor-C), a selective receptor for lymphatic vessel growth factors, is a neo angiogenic factor. The same applies to b-FGF (basic fibroblast growth factor) synthesised by the endothelial cells of abnormal lymphatic vessels [20, 22].

c.2. Evolution, clinical forms :

The severity of MLK depends essentially on the type and location of the disease [20].

Macrocystic lymphatic malformations are the most common MLKs (around 90%). They tend to develop in relapses

inflammatory response to intercurrent infection or trauma [20].

Intracystic haemorrhagic transformation is a classic complication. The swelling is painful, erythematous, warm and compressive. Some large MLKs have a potentially dangerous mediastinal extension. The actual size of the tumour is often underestimated despite radiological evaluation [20].

Some cysts progress suddenly during childhood and puberty, when the malformation reaches its final size. Rarely, they regress spontaneously during the fibrous healing of an inflammatory or infectious outbreak [20].

Microcystic lymphatic malformations are generally without clinical repercussions other than aesthetic, occasionally complicating inflammatory episodes, superinfections or bleeding [20].

Some locations present functional and vital damage:

- Oral MLK is responsible for macroglossia, mandibular deformity due to bone infiltration, and even prognathism, accompanied by disorders of the dental articulation. Oozing, bleeding and superinfection of oral vesicles are common;
- Laryngeal MLK is at risk of respiratory distress and dysphagia;
- orbital MLK causes visual impairment [20].

c.3 Imaging :

Their characteristics are similar to venous malformations. Their imaging is based on a combination of ultrasound and MRI, the latter being reserved for infiltrating locations, particularly craniocervical and mediastinal, and for preoperative mapping. However, there are a number of special features [20]:

- Macrocystic and microcystic forms: in the microcystic forms, the cysts are very small (submillimetre) and the fleshy component (cyst walls) predominates over the fluid contingent.
- Imaging reveals a rather compact mass with :
  - presence of fine vessels in the cyst walls;
  - frequent presence of liquid-debris levels within cysts

Evidence of intra-lesional haemorrhage;

- absence of dilated or tortuous veins in the vicinity [2].

Ultrasound :

Macrocystic lymphomas are multilocular with partitions of varying thickness. The contents are generally anechoic but become echogenic in the event of bleeding or infection (Figure 10). Microcystic lymphomas appear echogenic because of the numerous interfaces they cross [23].

MRI :

The ML show a hypointense signal in T1 and a hyperintense signal in T2 with hypointense trabeculae corresponding to the fibrous partitions. A hyperintense signal in T1 and liquid-liquid levels may be observed in the case of haemorrhagic or lipid content (Figure 11). Unlike MV, the lumen does not take up contrast [23].

Other imaging methods :

Arteriography, phlebography and lymphography do not contribute to the diagnosis.

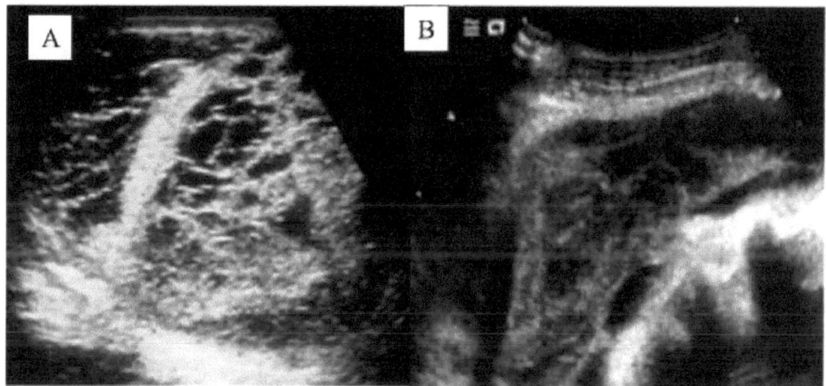

Figure 10: Multi-compartment cystic mass (A) complicated by an intracystic haematoma (B) [24].

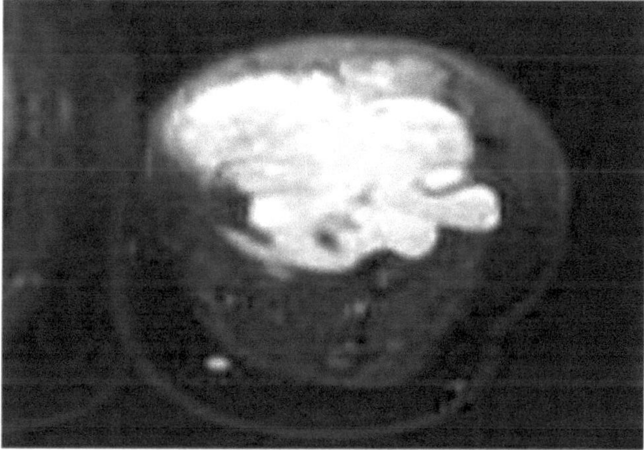

Figure 11: MRI T2 sequence, lymphatic malformation of the left arm [23].

1.6.2. Rapid-flow vascular malformation

a. Arteriovenous malformations :

Arteriovenous malformations (AVMs) are the most dangerous malformations because they are haemodynamically active, with sometimes dramatic worsening. They are difficult to treat.

There are two categories:

- arteriovenous fistula, congenital or post-traumatic, consisting of a shunt between an artery and a vein;
- The arteriovenous malformation itself comprises a nidus with multiple arterial and venous shunts.

These superficial AVMs can involve all areas of the skin without gender predominance, and it is important to make the diagnosis clinically in order to avoid untimely or inappropriate procedures which could lead to a secondary increase in the size of the malformation [25].

a.1. Clinical characteristics

AVMs are rare and serious vascular malformations. Lesions are present at birth in 40% to 60% of infants and appear in childhood in around 30% of cases. They are most often located in the cephalic region (Figure 12), preferentially affecting the head and neck, possibly for embryological reasons [26].

In 1990, the International Society for the Study of Vascular Anomalies (ISSVA) defined a severity scale, also known as "Schobinger staging", to classify AVMs into different stages of increasing severity [12] :

- **Stage I** is a dormant stage in which the AVM is asymptomatic and quiescent. During this stage, the angioma may be completely invisible or take on the appearance of an erythematous macule simulating a flat angioma or involutional haemangioma. The diagnosis is sometimes corrected by palpation of a thrill, auscultation of a murmur, or even the mere perception of an increase in local heat, which raise suspicions of a high-flow malformation. This stage is most frequently observed in childhood and into adolescence, but may persist throughout life [12].
- **Stage II** is an expansion stage. The physical and hormonal changes inherent in puberty and even pregnancy are often described as the main factors in the development of this stage. However, certain accidental or iatrogenic traumas, including laser treatments, feeder artery ligatures, incomplete arterial embolisation or partial excision of the malformation, can also precipitate the transition to this stage. More rarely, the condition is aggravated by thrombotic or infectious episodes. Vascular lesions darken and increase in size, distorting the integument and invading deeper structures. Diagnosis is made on the basis of the same, often more significant, signs as at the initial stage [26] ;
- **Stage III** corresponds to the stage of destruction where, in addition to the characteristics of stage II, there are integumentary alterations such as spontaneous necrosis and chronic ulcerations, which are a source of pain and bleeding. This skin destruction is sometimes also associated with bone lysis [26].
- **stage IV** is characterised by the appearance of heart failure due to poor tolerance of the increase in blood flow within the malformation, resulting in haemodistortion. This stage is in fact extremely rare, affecting only 1 to 2% of patients [26].

a.2. Pathophysiology

Unlike arteriovenous fistulas, where there is only a single shunt zone between an

artery and a vein, AVMs are composed of multiple shunts made up of arteriovenous structures forming a nidus fed by several arteries and draining into several veins. This aspect largely explains the therapeutic difficulties encountered when attempting to treat these malformations. The genesis of AVMs is currently explained by a defect in the regression of primitive retiform plexuses at an early stage of embryonic development. This theory explains why AVMs are more frequent in the head and neck region, mainly affecting the cheeks and ears, which have the highest "surface to volume" ratio during the embryonic period [26].
Hypotheses concerning the biological mechanisms of AVM formation currently favour a deficit in apoptosis pathways and dysregulation of vascular differentiation signals. Furthermore, although most AVMs occur sporadically and are not hereditary, it has recently been shown that certain syndromes such as capillary and arteriovenous malformation syndrome are directly linked to a genetic mutation [26].

a.3. Clinical diagnosis

The diagnosis of AVM is most often suspected clinically in the presence of a red cutaneous and/or subcutaneous swelling with signs of haemodynamic activity: increased local heat, thrill, auscultatory murmur or murmur detected by portable Doppler. Other conditions, signs of a more advanced stage, should also lead to a diagnosis: significant or unusual pain in the angioma, episodes of bleeding or ulceration, localised muscle or bone hypertrophy reflecting regional hypervascularisation. The main differential diagnoses discussed in the early stages are a low-flow vascular malformation, a haemangioma, which also shows signs of haemodynamic activity during its growth phase, or even neoplasia, particularly vascular angiosarcoma. When localised to the lower limb, the malformation may also resemble Kaposi's sarcoma [23].

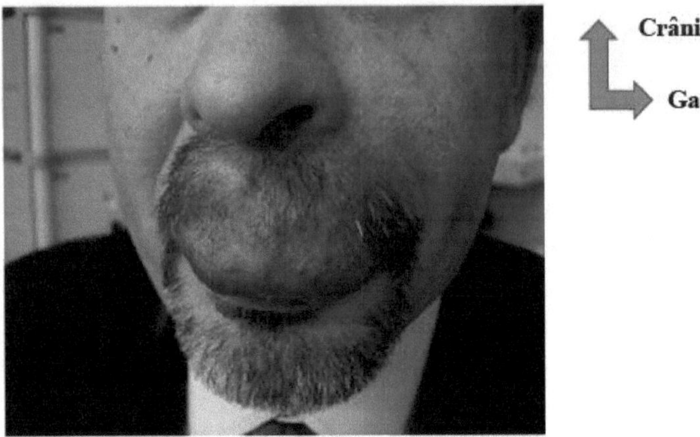

Figure 12: Arteriovenous malformation of the upper lip: red, warm, throbbing swelling [2].

a.4. Histology: [15]

The lesion is poorly defined. It is made up of vessels of very varied size, ovoid or slightly irregular in shape, regularly dispersed in the tissues. Their walls are often relatively thin compared with the diameter of the lumen, and vary in thickness from one point of the circumference to another.

It is best analysed by staining elastic tissue. Some vessels have an arterial or venous structure. Others are difficult to classify, with an almost absent elastic architecture or an intermediate appearance between artery and vein.

Direct communications between arterial vessels and veins are observed. AVMs also have a capillary component, which is sometimes significant, and may have a lobulated appearance somewhat reminiscent of infantile haemangiomas. In other cases, the appearance may be that of an angiolipoma, as in the case of vascular tumours and malformations, anatomopathological classification and imaging 277.

Mitoses may be observed in the capillary component.

In rare cases, there are dilated vessels on the surface with very thin walls, which may suggest cystic fibrosis. However, they never form such a complex, anastomosing network or dissect the tissues. Finally, AVMs are often associated with fairly significant collagen fibrosis.

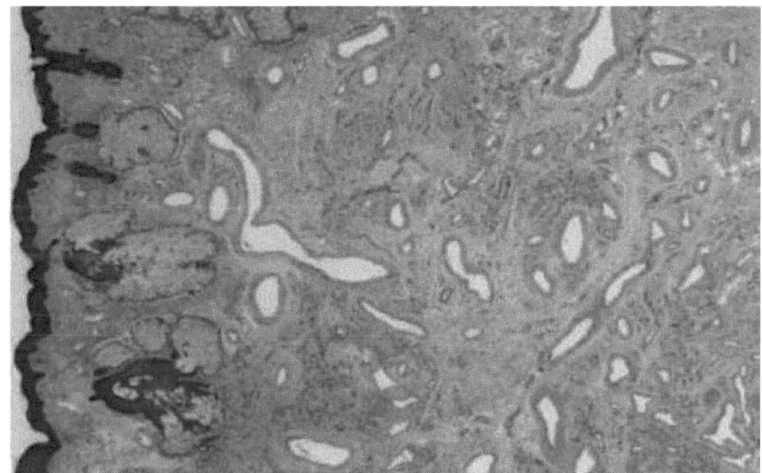

Figure 13: Nasal arteriovenous malformation: presence of thick-walled vessels of a thickness proportional to their lumen in abnormal numbers, distributed in the dermis. Note the presence of a component of small vessels [27].

a.5. Biological characteristics :

It is recommended that a haemostasis test be carried out in cases of venous involvement, due to the risk of coagulopathy, particularly in cases of extensive venous malformations [28].

Plasma D-dimer, platelet and fibrinogen levels should be consulted, and the date of sampling noted. Plasma D-dimer levels and fibrinogen are recommended as part of the initial work-up for the management of extensive extra-truncular venous malformations (recommendation level 1 C, International Union of Phlebology consensus 2013) [28].

Since localised intravascular coagulation phenomena are possible, it is recommended that the following assays be performed when monitoring extensive or high-risk venous malformations, or as a pre-therapeutic measure for invasive procedures:

- Blood count: haemoglobin, platelets,
- Quantitative D-dimer,
- Fibrinogen,
- Fibrin degradation product or fibrin monomers,
- TP, TCA [8].

a.6 Imaging :

Radiological assessment is essential not only to confirm the diagnosis but also to define the extent of the lesion and its haemodynamic characteristics, which largely determine the prognosis and treatment options [26].

Doppler ultrasound and magnetic resonance imaging (MRI) are the 2 radiological examinations that complement each other in characterising AVMs [26].

Doppler ultrasound

It is often performed as a first-line procedure. It often confirms the diagnosis of AVM. Pulsed Doppler measures resistance indexes and establishes a comparative evaluation of flow rates (in extremity forms) as well as identifying fistula points. It is also used to monitor the disease and detect sub-clinical flare-ups. By its very nature, this examination is operator-dependent. It is also limited when lesions are deep, not easily accessible and/or located close to or infiltrating bone or air structures [29,30].

Although it does not offer the same ability to visualise flows in real time as Doppler ultrasound, MRI is also a very useful examination for exploring AVMs. It offers an optimal overview of the vascular structures of the malformation and its anatomical relationships with adjacent and deep organs. It provides an objective view of the rapid flow, which is often accompanied by areas devoid of signal, reflecting rapid, turbulent blood flow. Flow rates can also be explored using gradient-echo mode, the equivalent of flow-weighted images [29,30].

The echodoppler (ED) is the basic examination for any suspected vascular anomaly. In the paediatric population, this test is even more useful, as it does not require sedation (as is sometimes the case for MRI, which requires strict immobility, which is difficult to obtain without sedation, depending on the age of the child). ED is therefore often the only complementary examination in children who do not present any signs of seriousness, until they are old enough to undergo other investigations [29,30].

B-mode analysis can be used to differentiate vascular tumours from vascular malformations and to determine in which plane the malformation is located (subcutaneous, muscular) [29,30].

Doppler analysis can differentiate between "slow flow" and "fast flow" malformations with the presence of an arteriovenous shunt (AVS). It can sometimes be used to identify the main afferent artery and the draining vein(s). The calibre of the afferent artery (increased upstream of the AVM) is one of the important parameters for monitoring AVMs. The Doppler spectrum is characterised by rapid systolo-diastolic flow at low resistance (high peak systolic velocity and permanent diastolic flow, reflecting the shunt effect). Objective measurement of flow (ml/min) in the main artery upstream of the

The flow of the AVM is compared with the flow of the same contralateral artery when this is possible, and makes it possible to estimate the flow attributable to the AVM. In terms of venous flow, the drainage veins present an abnormally pulsatile and "arterialised" spectrum [29,30].

These characteristics are used for both initial diagnosis and follow-up, representing objective elements in the evaluation of the evolution of the malformation or the effect of any embolisation. The main limitation of ED exploration is its operator-dependent nature and the need for specific expertise on the part of the vascular physician with an integrative view of the clinic so that the best management can then be discussed at a multidisciplinary consultation [29].

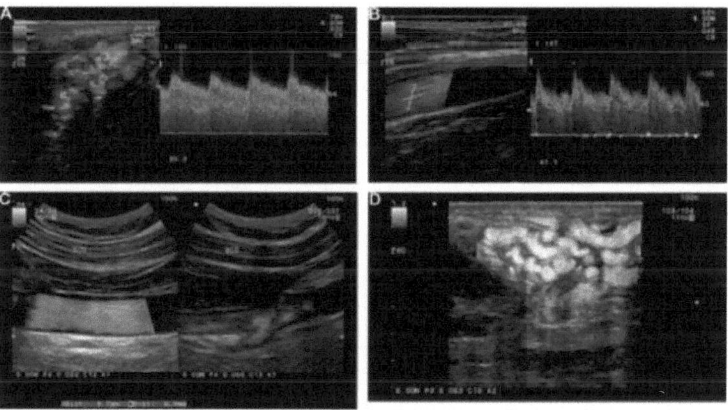

Figure 14: Rapid systolo-diastolic flow at low resistance (A) within the AVM and (B) within the afferent artery. C. Difference in diameter between the afferent artery [30].

MRI :

It also identifies areas of haemorrhage or thrombosis manifested by a T1-weighted hypersignal. The presence of a fatty signal within the lesion, muscle atrophy and the absence of peri-lesional oedema rule out the differential diagnosis of a tumour. On the other hand, it is sometimes possible to rectify the diagnosis when faced with a lesion that is vascular in the periphery but solid in the centre, which should prompt discussion of a surgical biopsy. A general anaesthetic is sometimes required for this to be carried out correctly in young children. MRI is often a necessary adjunct to ultrasound exploration. MRI can be used to assess the morphology of the AVM as a whole and to estimate its extent and impact on the deep planes and neighbouring structures (muscle and bone invasion, etc.). Dynamic sequences can be used to highlight the precise location of the arteriovenous shunt(s) [26].

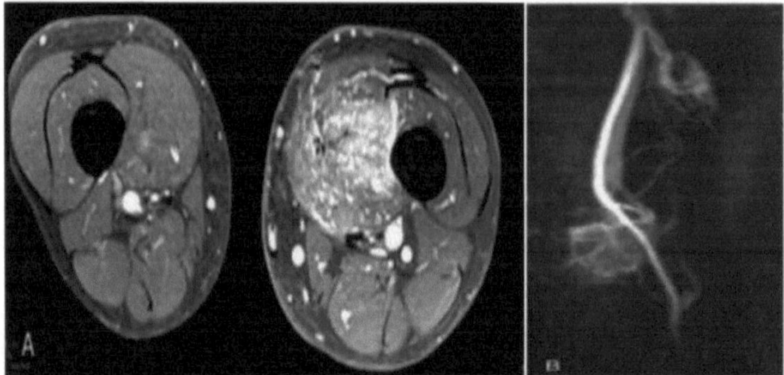

Figure 15: AVM of the left thigh

A. T2 MRI, Axial sections of the thighs showing an intramuscular hypervascularised structure of the thigh G;

B. Angio-MRI reconstruction of the G thigh showing the nidus fed by the superficial femoral artery; early venous enhancement is evidence of the arteriovenous shunt [31].

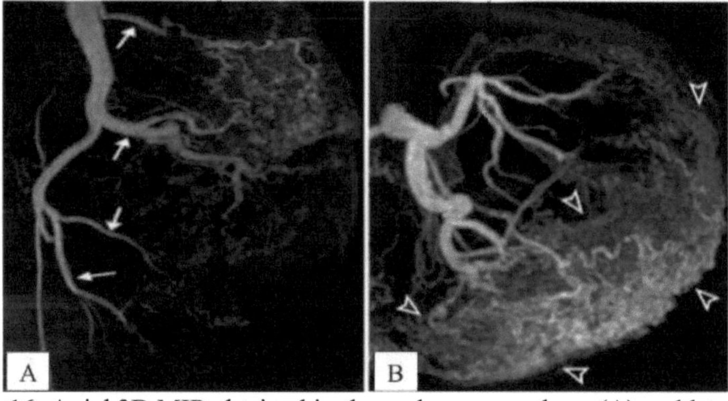

Figure 16: Axial 3D MIP obtained in the early venous phase (A) and late phase (B) showing a femoral AVM with a nidus [32].

CT :

It is performed with injection of contrast medium, visualises the malformation and is useful for determining its skeletal or visceral extension. It is intrinsically limited for exploring soft tissue and blood flow.

In addition, its ionising properties make it difficult to repeat the examinations necessary for monitoring children. For these reasons, this examination is not currently the preferred option for exploring AVMs [26].

Arteriography :

It was most often necessary for the initial assessment of the disease, and advances in MRI often obviate the need for diagnostic arteriography. It is essential for planning aggressive treatment by embolisation or surgery. The

arteriography technique involves percutaneous arterial puncture, generally in the femoral artery, with insertion of a catheter. It must include selective catheterisation of the various arterial branches [26].
The radiological signs are dilatation of the afferent arteries confluent at the heart of the nidus, excluding adjacent territories, and very rapid circulation with immediate venous return at the arterial time of the arteriogram.
Although this examination is still essential for therapeutic procedures, its exploratory function is currently being superseded by MRI angiography, which is increasingly better at characterising the feeder arteries and drainage veins, but with a definition that is currently inferior to that of true catheter angiography [26].

Echocardiography :

This examination is carried out systematically when a high-flow AVM is diagnosed. It is used to look for any cardiac repercussions, which would indicate the need for interventional management [8].

a.7. Therapeutic management

The management of AVMs is problematic because the risk of decompensation of the malformation is major. Incomplete treatment almost systematically leads to recurrence and often worsening of the disease [23].
This is why, except in exceptional cases, invasive treatment is usually avoided during the quiescent stage of the disease. This abstention from treatment is accompanied by preventive advice aimed at reducing the risk of progression [23].
The measures usually recommended are abstention from sports or professional activities involving a risk of violent or repeated trauma. Careful clinical and radiological monitoring of the AVM is carried out [23].
The therapeutic decision is most often taken on the basis of clinical criteria, rather than the radiological evolutionary profile [23].
There are two types of treatment:

❖ **Endovascular treatment :**

This treatment is indicated in adults because many of the risks are related to trauma or vascular immaturity [23].
The main indications are: an extreme increase in pain, the appearance of an ulceration, an AVM that has become haemorrhagic, or significant and rapid extension of the malformation. On the other hand, a minor flare-up, for example secondary to trauma, may only be temporary and regress in a few months. It is therefore not always an indication for immediate surgery [23].
In these difficult cases, it is sometimes necessary to take a wait-and-see approach, and organise even more careful follow-up with photographic and

Doppler reassessments [23].

❖ **Conventional treatment :**

When the decision is taken, the operation often combines embolisation and complete surgical removal of the AVM, depending on the location; the more superficial the AVM, the greater the need for skin removal [26].

The main exception to this rule is the exceptional case of symptomatic treatment, of a bleed for example, where an endovascular procedure alone is sufficient [26].

Embolisation reduces intra-operative bleeding, in preparation for improved surgical resection. Proximal ligation or embolisation of the afferent arteries is ineffective and dangerous. They close off the access routes to the malformation and increase its network of collaterals. Several embolisation techniques have been discussed [26].

The endovascular route is always to be preferred, but is sometimes limited by the impossibility of correctly reaching the area to be embolised. Direct puncture of the malformation, carried out after angiographic identification, provides faster and more reliable access to the area to be treated, but carries the risk of extravasation or foreign body reaction within the AVM [26].

Many sclerosing products are used. Ethanol remains the most effective molecule, but its toxicity limits injectable doses to 1ml/kg of weight in adults, with a lower maximum dose in children (generally less than 0.5ml/kg in older children). Biological glues and microparticles are also frequently used [26].

When it is decided, surgical removal is radical, of the carcinological type. It is sometimes preceded by the insertion of skin expanders to optimise reconstruction. Careful dissection spares the venous returns as much as possible. The technique of reconstructive surgery is discussed on a case-by-case basis [26].

b. Syndromic forms :

AVMs are sometimes only part of an underlying disease and are then associated with systemic abnormalities.

Several syndromes have been identified. Early recognition of these syndromes is a necessary step, as the abnormalities associated with them determine the prognosis and influence treatment [26].

b.1. Bonnet-Duchaume-White syndrome (Wyburn-Mason)

Bonnet-Duchaume-Blanc (BDB) syndrome was first reported by Bonnet and his team in 1937, and then reproduced in English-language literature by Wyburn 6 years later [26].

This non-hereditary syndrome combines mesencephalic involvement, an ipsilateral retinal malformation and a quiescent stage AVM, sometimes inconstant, which may be located either in a trigeminal territory or in a centrofacial position. Clinical neurological signs include progressive focal neurological deficits depending on the territory in which the malformation is located, epilepsy, headache and, more rarely, psychomotor retardation [26].

These symptoms indicate cerebral suffering due to venous congestion or haemorrhage. Maxillofacial lesions may be present, causing facial deformities, alterations in maxillofacial bone growth and, in the case of intraosseous maxillomandibular lesions, serious oral haemorrhage. Visual symptoms result from arteriovenous malformations of the retina and depend on the size and location of the malformations (retina, optic nerve, chiasma) [26].

BDB is the result of an anomaly in organogenesis. The link between these lesions of the same angioarchitectural nature, but of different location, is explained by the regionalised origin of the cells of the vascular walls of the cephalic region and their migration. Retinal vascular malformation is identified by fundus examination [26].

MRI is used to diagnose and characterise all lesions. Cerebral arteriography identifies the possibility of embolisation, which is particularly problematic in this location [26].

b.2. Parkes-Weber syndrome

Parkes-Weber syndrome or angio-osteohypertrophic syndrome (AOH) is a congenital bone vascular syndrome characterised by the presence of an arteriovenous malformation in a limb that affects bone metabolism by stimulating elongation during growth [26].

Overgrowth affects a single bone (mainly the femur or tibia) or, in some cases, the whole limb. Limb length discrepancy (LLD) becomes evident between infancy and adolescence. The skin involvement of Parkes-Weber syndrome is an AVM, most often in the quiescent stage, but other manifestations such as superficial vein dilatation, lymphatic involvement and limb enlargement are frequently observed [26].

Although Parkes-Weber syndrome is generally sporadic, autosomal dominant inheritance has been observed in a small number of families. Diagnosis is based on clinical examination, radiographs (preferably in the upright position to assess MLD and to study any changes in bone structure), and various techniques for mapping the malformation [26].

The differential diagnosis includes venous dysplasia, lymphoedema and bone tumours. During the growth period in childhood, treatment of AVM is aimed at correcting MLD. Orthopaedic procedures stop bone elongation during the growth period or correct MLD in adults. When decided, epiphysiodesis is performed using the least invasive technique possible, usually percutaneous, at the risk of aggravating the deformity. Elongation of the contralateral limb using the Ilizarov technique can be envisaged in adults [26].

b.3. Capillary and arteriovenous malformation syndrome

The capillary and arteriovenous malformation syndrome is a recently described hereditary syndrome associating a high-flow vascular anomaly with a capillary malformation [26].

It results from mutations in the RASA1 gene encoding a signalling protein for growth factor receptors (p120-rasGAP), involved in the proliferation, migration and survival of endothelial cells. Arteriovenous malformations are located in the skin, bone, muscle or brain. Capillary malformation is often characterised by a peripheral pale halo. Borderline forms with Parkes-Weber syndrome have been described [26].

b.4. Cobb syndrome

Cobb syndrome or cutaneous-meningospinal angiomatosis is a rare, non-hereditary syndrome defined by the association of cutaneous and medullary arteriovenous malformations of the same metamer or spinal segment. There may also be bone and/or muscle involvement. The AVM is most often in the quiescent stage. Exceptionally, it may be replaced by angiokeratoma, angiolipoma or lymphangioma type lesions. This syndrome frequently becomes symptomatic in early adolescence, often following the appearance of the first neurological symptoms, testifying to a phenomenon of vascular flight, nerve compression, venous hypertension or haemorrhage [26].

These neurological symptoms vary in severity from transient sensory and/or motor disorders to sudden spastic quadriplegia. They also depend on the metamerism affected. Other less specific signs are suggestive: headache, meningeal syndrome or sphincter disorders. Neurological involvement is the most serious aspect of this syndrome, and it is important to recognise it early in the case of any metameric angioma that may indicate an underlying spinal arteriovenous malformation. The course is unpredictable, and lesions may remain asymptomatic for a long time [26].

1.7.Differential diagnosis

The differential diagnosis of these malformations poses a real diagnostic problem with vascular lesions of tumour origin in children [24].

1.7.1. Infantile haemangioma

It is the most common tumour in infants (10%), with a clear predominance of females, especially in severe forms (sex ratio: 5 girls/1 boy). It usually appears after a few days or weeks of life. In 95% of cases it regresses spontaneously without sequelae; therapeutic abstention is the rule [24].

There are three clinical types:

- the tuberous or superficial form corresponds to a red, prominent spot with an irregular surface and sharp edges, commonly known as a "strawberry" angioma;
- the subcutaneous form (affecting the deep dermis) takes the form of a swelling with a firm, elastic consistency, warm but not beating, raising slightly bluish or pinkish healthy skin;

The mixed form combines the two aspects: the tuberous part develops first and the deep part appears a few months later, overhanging the first with a bluish halo [24].

The superficial form regresses before the subcutaneous form [26].

The term "immature" underlines the triphasic evolutionary potential [24].

The natural history is stereotyped. A phase of rapid growth (in surface area and volume) between the first two months and 8^{e} months is followed by a period of stabilisation, then a slow phase of involution over several months or even years (2 to 12 years) [24].

Sequelae sometimes persist: extensive cutaneous haemangiomas may leave a telangiectatic scar, while subcutaneous or mixed haemangiomas leave distended and wrinkled skin [24].

Exceptionally, the functional or vital prognosis is threatened. Close monitoring is required during the critical phase of the first three months, as there is no way of predicting a severe form in the neonatal period [24].

1.7.2. Histology

Haemangiomas correspond to a proliferation of endothelial cells, a cell mass that feeds and drains through vascular neo-channels. Endothelial cells express certain proteins such as GLUT1 (also found in placental endothelial cells) [24].

They are not present in vascular malformations or congenital haemangiomas [24].

1.7.3. Clinical presentation and complications

They are usually single and do not exceed 3 cm in size. Whatever the morphology of immature haemangiomas in infants, they are seen in all locations, but preferentially in the cervicofacial region (60%) [23].

Some of these localisations are particular, such as the haemangioma of the tip of the nose called "Cyrano" or the labial haemangioma "tapir" [23].

1.7.4. Periorificial haemangiomas (perioral, palpebral, auricular, anogenital):

Orbito-palpebral haemangiomas cause amblyopia through reduction of the palpebral slit, compression of the eyeball or infiltration of the orbital cone and oculomotor muscles [24].

Labial localisation hinders sucking and weight gain in infants.

Haemangiomas of the external auditory canal are obstructive and cause

superinfections (otitis externa and otitis media) [24].
Similarly, nasal wing haemangiomas cause locoregional superinfections [24].
Ano-genital haemangiomas ulcerate on contact with the nappies and frequently become necrotic [24].
Cervical haemangiomas sometimes extend into the tracheolaryngeal tract, causing dyspnoea and requiring emergency treatment [24].
A classic complication of haemangioma with a tuberous component is necrosis. Whether iatrogenic or spontaneous in origin, these ulcerations are very painful, a source of superinfection and bleeding, sometimes life-threatening. They leave an unsightly scar [24].

1.7.5. Visceral haemangiomas :

They are rare and should not be systematically sought in the presence of a superficial location, as the vast majority will regress in the same way as cutaneous forms. They are more frequent in diffuse miliary cutaneous haemangiomatosis [24].
Hepatic localization, which can be voluminous, is manifested by hepatomegaly, haemodynamic disorders and even cardiac failure [24].

1.7.6. Extensive haemangiomas in surface or thickness :

They represent significant aesthetic and functional damage. Heart failure is more frequently observed in this group [24].

1.7.7. Specific syndromes :

Segmental haemangiomas are frequently associated with extracutaneous abnormalities [24].
The PHACES syndrome includes anomalies of the posterior intracranial fossa (Dandy-Walker syndrome), facial haemangioma, encephalic arterial malformations, aortic coarctation, congenital cardiac anomalies, ocular anomalies and sternal anomalies [24]. A urogenital haemangioma is a segmental anomaly of the nappy area (lumbosacral, gluteal or perineal region) [24].
It is the marker of a dysraphia affecting to varying degrees the lumbosacral spine, the terminal medullary cone, the genitourinary organs and the anal region. Known as the "PELVIS-SACRAL" syndrome, its diagnosis is delayed or difficult because of its unusual clinical presentation: macular, telangiectatic or livedoid [24].

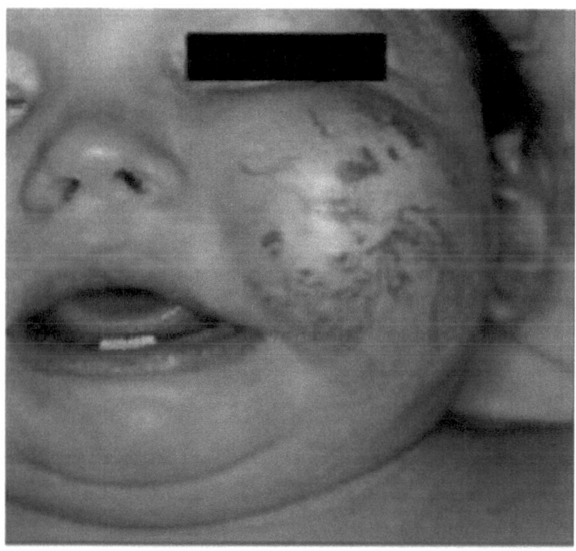

Figure 17: Infantile haemangioma of the left cheek, mixed form [2].

1.8.Other childhood vascular tumours

1.8.1. Congenital haemangiomas :

They are exceptional and present differently from infantile haemangiomas. They are fully developed in utero and do not grow after birth. Histologically different from previously described haemangiomas, they have large veins and lymphatic vessels within them[24].

Their preferential location affects the scalp or the limbs close to a large joint. Some will rapidly involute within 6 to 14 months after birth and are termed RICH (rapidly involuting congenital hemangioma) and others will be non-involuting, termed NICH (non-involuting congenital hemangioma) [24].

RICH can be clinically alarming, highly vascularised and resembling a malignant tumour requiring diagnostic biopsy. NICH is clinically less impressive, resembling a relapsing infantile haemangioma [24].

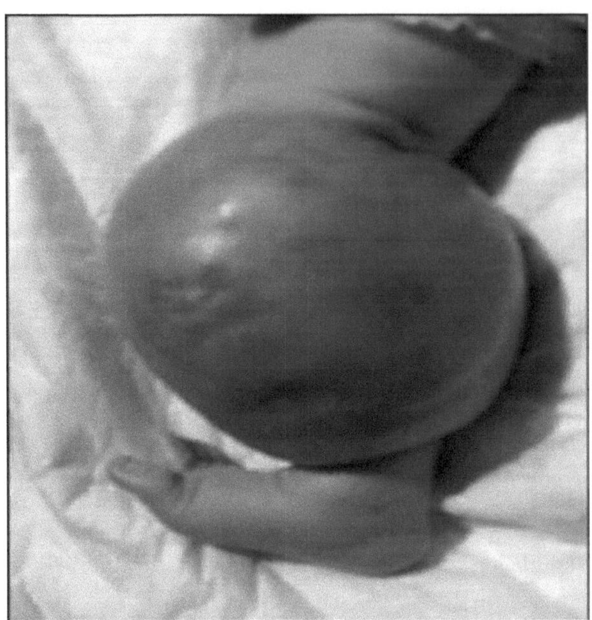

Figure 18: Very large rapidly involuting congenital hemangioma (RICH) [24].

1.8.2. Tufted haemangiomas :

They are rare, usually acquired but may be congenital, and progress slowly. They appear as red patches or a prominent purplish tumour [24].

Histologically, it is a capillary dispersion in small clumps, surrounded by a crescent-shaped vessel with an empty lumen. These haemangiomas may be associated with Kasabach-Merritt syndrome, with a pseudo-inflammatory transformation and the appearance of sequestration thrombocytopenia [24].

1.8.3. Kaposiform haemangioendothelioma

This rare vascular tumour appears as a nodular infiltration of the subcutaneous tissue. It is very often associated with Kasabach-Merritt syndrome.

It is clinically similar to tufted haemangioma (although the primary lesions are more infiltrative) and they are currently considered to be a single entity [24].

Kasabach Merritt syndrome or "infantile tumour syndrome". This rare pseudo-inflammatory transformation, associated with major thrombocytopenia and drug-induced coagulopathy, affected classic infantile haemangiomas indiscriminately. However, haemangiomas at risk do not express the glut-1 marker and are therefore associated with vascular tumours of the tufted haemangioma or kaposiform haemangioendothelioma type [24].

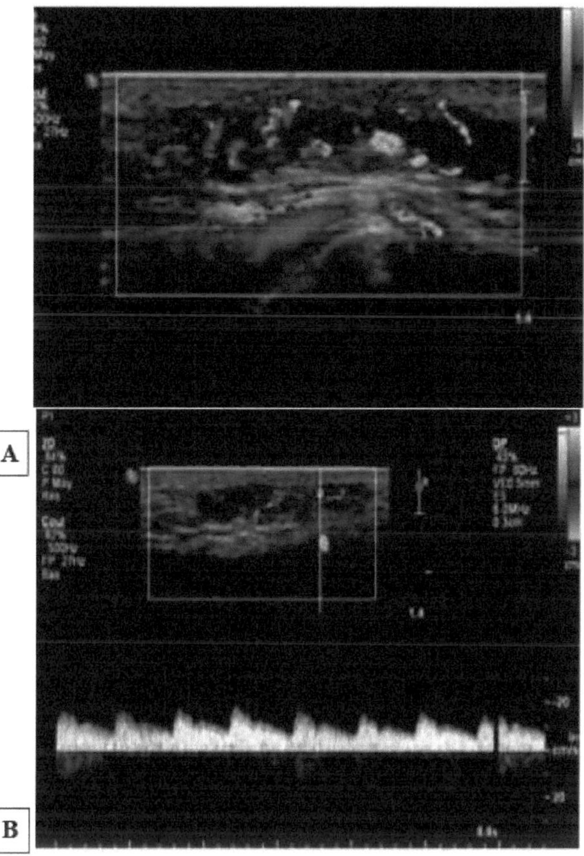

Figure 19: Infantile hemangioma [24].

swelling delimited by hypervascularisation

A) Low resistance arterial flow with resistance index close to 0.5.

CHAPTER 2

2. OUR STUDY

2.1.Type and period of study

This was a descriptive study carried out in December 2022 of a case of arteriovenous malformation diagnosed in the medical imaging department and managed by the thoracic and cardiovascular surgery department.

2.2.Setting and place of study

Our study was carried out in the medical imaging department of Mali Hospital. This hospital is a 3eme referral hospital structure established by Law N° 010 of 20 May 2010. It is a product of Sino-Malian cooperation, inaugurated in 2010 and opened its doors in September 2011. According to law N° 10010 of 20 May 2010, Mali's hospital is a public hospital (EPH). It has legal personality and financial autonomy. Its mission is to participate in the implementation of national health policy. To this end, it is responsible for

- Diagnose and treat the sick and injured, pregnant women and children;
- Handling emergencies and referrals;
- Participate in the initial and continuing training of healthcare professionals;
- Conducting research in the medical field.

It is located on the right bank of the River Niger in the Missabougou neighbourhood in Commune VI of the Bamako district.

- **Infrastructure :**

The department has a patient reception area.

Three X-ray rooms, including (01) a remote-controlled room and (02) two bone and lung X-ray rooms, a digital room for image processing, a scanner room, an MRI room, a mammography room, an ultrasound room, an interpretation room, an on-call room, two toilets, five offices and a waiting room.

- **Department staff :**

Six radiologists, one of whom is Chinese, one ultrasound technician, seven (07) medical assistants, one senior health technician and one (01) secretary,
a labourer.

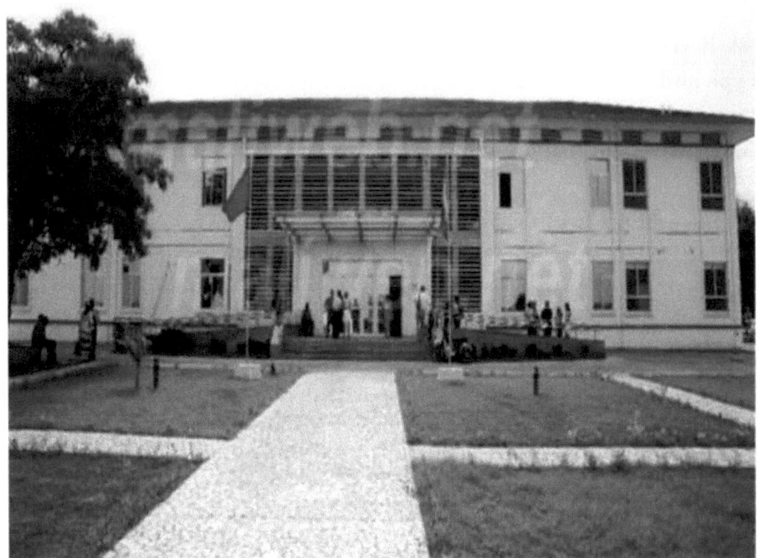

Figure 20: Photograph of Mali Hospital (front view)

2.3.Observation :

A 15-day-old female newborn (born on 07 December 2022), the first sibling of a full-term pregnancy well monitored by a midwife and an euto-cic delivery. At birth, she weighed 3600 grams. She had no particular family history. This newborn was referred to us (22 December 2022) by the paediatrics department for a Doppler ultrasound scan of the right elbow, for a congenital mass of the right elbow.

On clinical examination, inspection revealed a raised, well-defined, bluish mass, erythematous in places, on the posteromedial aspect of the right elbow. Palpation revealed a warm, pulsatile mass with thrills. Auscultation of the swelling revealed a murmur. There was no bleeding or ulceration of the mass (Figure 21).

The biological work-up was normal overall.

There were no associated malformations.

The echodoppler, performed using a 12 MHz linear probe on a GE LOGIQ7 ultrasound machine, revealed poorly limited vascular dilatations of multiple fast-flow arteriovenous fistulas within the periarticular mass of the right elbow (Figure 23).

To better characterise this mass, we performed an angioscan of the right upper limb (December 22, 2022). We used a Siemens 16-slice scanner with an acquisition console and two syngovia processing consoles.

An angioscan protocol was carried out with millimetric acquisition, axial slices in a soft tissue filter. After a period without injection of the iodinated contrast product in search of a possible haemorrhagic complication, arterial and venous acquisition was performed after intravenous (IV) injection of 10ml of 350mg iodine (OMNIPAQUE). Coronal and sagittal reconstructions in MPR, MIP and 3D for better exposure of the vessels were performed. The CT scan showed a heterogeneous, hyperdense, homogeneous, well-defined tissue mass (49UH) of the right elbow with no calcification or associated haemorrhage prior to contrast injection.

After injection of contrast (angioscan protocol), vascular dilatations were noted with multiple subcutaneous arteriovenous shunts on the posteromedial aspect of the elbow, creating a mass (nidus) measuring 61x46mm. This mass was fed by the right brachial artery (arrow fig. 24 A) with an arteriovenous fistula between the latter and the homolateral basilic vein upstream of the mass (double-headed arrow fig. 24 A). It was drained by the homolateral basilic vein (yellow arrow fig.24B). The cephalic vein was slightly dilated with no arteriovenous fistula (arrowhead fig.24 B).

There were small arterial branches emanating from the brachial artery in the forearm (Figure 24 A).

The evolution was marked by a complication in the form of active bleeding (24 days later, 15 January 2023), prompting a visit to the emergency department. A pressure bandage with a tourniquet was applied for 15 minutes, which stopped the bleeding. After removal of the tourniquet, a pulsatile vascular dilatation of approximately 5/4 cm with a central ulcero-necrotic lesion was noted (Figure 22). There were no cardiopulmonary abnormalities. The diagnosis of a Schöbinger stage III arteriovenous malformation of the right elbow was made.

Open surgery was performed by the cardiovascular and thoracic surgery team, together with a radiologist and an intensive care anaesthetist (28 January 2023).

After general anaesthesia and rigorous asepsis, we made a 05cm incision upstream of the swelling on the inside of the right arm, followed by subcutaneous musculoaponeurotic dissection until the brachial artery was exposed and a 2ième fusiform incision removing the wound from which the fistula was bleeding.

Investigation revealed a right brachio-basilic arteriovenous fistula with an upstream dilated basilic vein and a multitude of subcutaneous veins under the swelling (Figure 25). We removed the arteriovenous communication using 6/0 prolene and removed the supply to the subcutaneous veins that had developed at the site of the artery using 3/0 prolene thread, then lined the cavity and carried out careful haemostasis. Afterwards, the subcutaneous veins were closed in 2 planes with 3/0 vicryl and the cutaneous veins with 2/0 skin suture. The incident

encountered during the operation was profuse bleeding of around 150cc, which was corrected by the transfusion of 300ml of whole blood. There were no accidents or immediate postoperative complications (Figure 26).
Histological examination of the surgical specimen revealed fibrous connective tissue interspersed with venules and arterioles that were sometimes connected and dilated without atypia. The surface was regular skin tissue compatible with an arteriovenous malformation. There were no tumour cells (Figure 27).
A follow-up angioscan was performed 07 months after surgery, demonstrating recurrence of the arteriovenous malformation drained by the basilic vein and fed by collateral branches of the brachial artery (Figure 28).

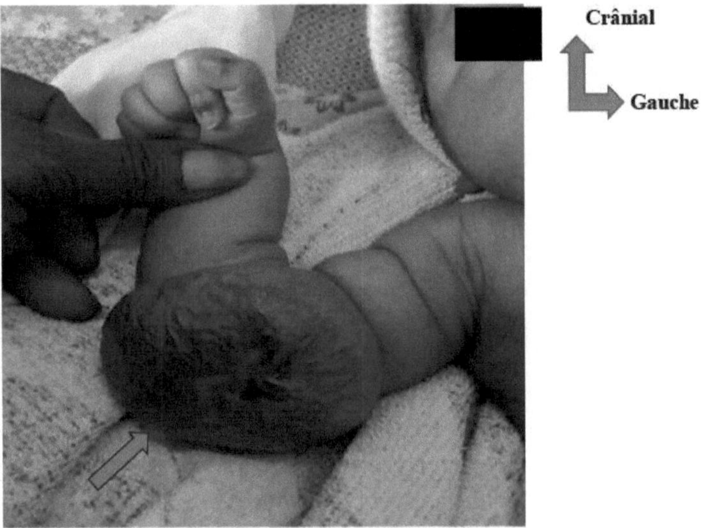

Figure 21: Image of the right elbow mass at D0 of birth (arrow).

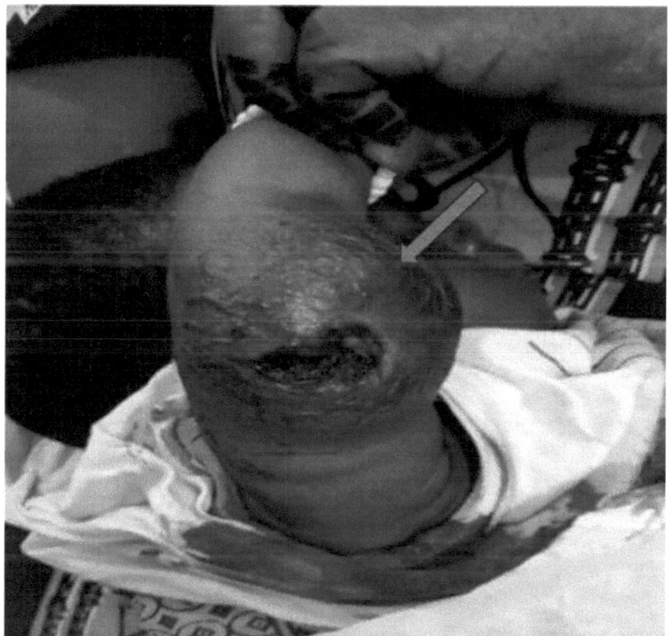

Figure 22: Image of ulceration of the right elbow mass (arrow) after active bleeding.

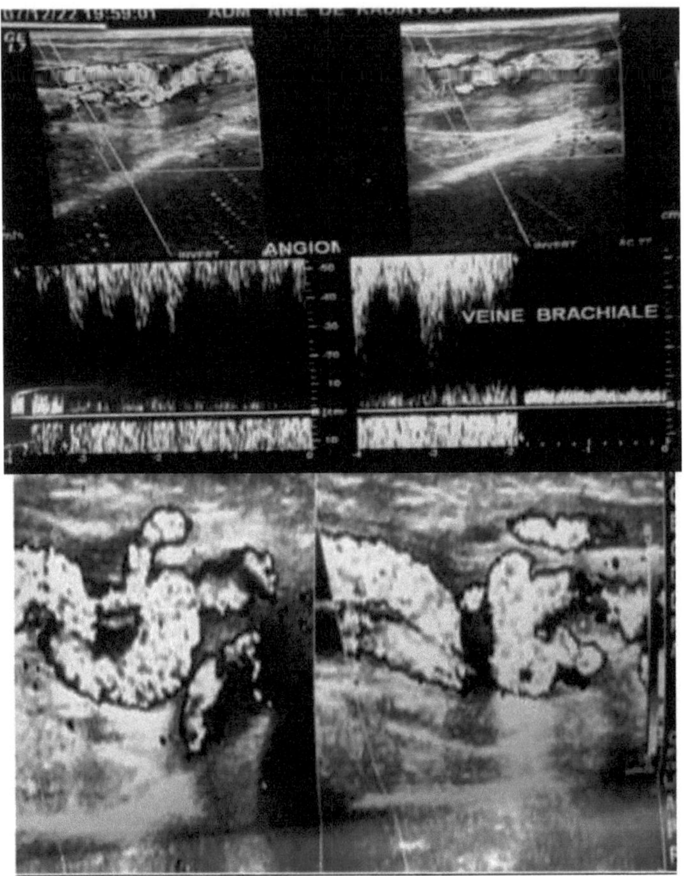

Figure 23: Vascular dilatation with diffuse colour Doppler coding and rapid arterial flow

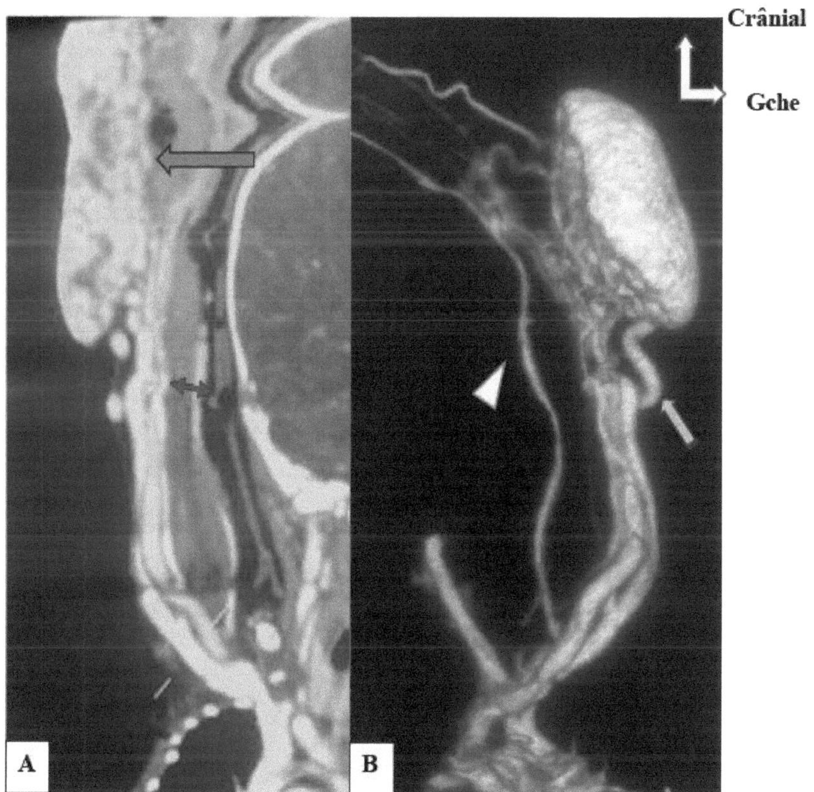

Figure 24: Angio-CT images of the right elbow AVM in coronal MIP reconstruction (A) and 3D (B) demonstrating vascular dilatation (arrow) with arteriovenous shunts between the brachial artery and basilic vein (arrowhead).

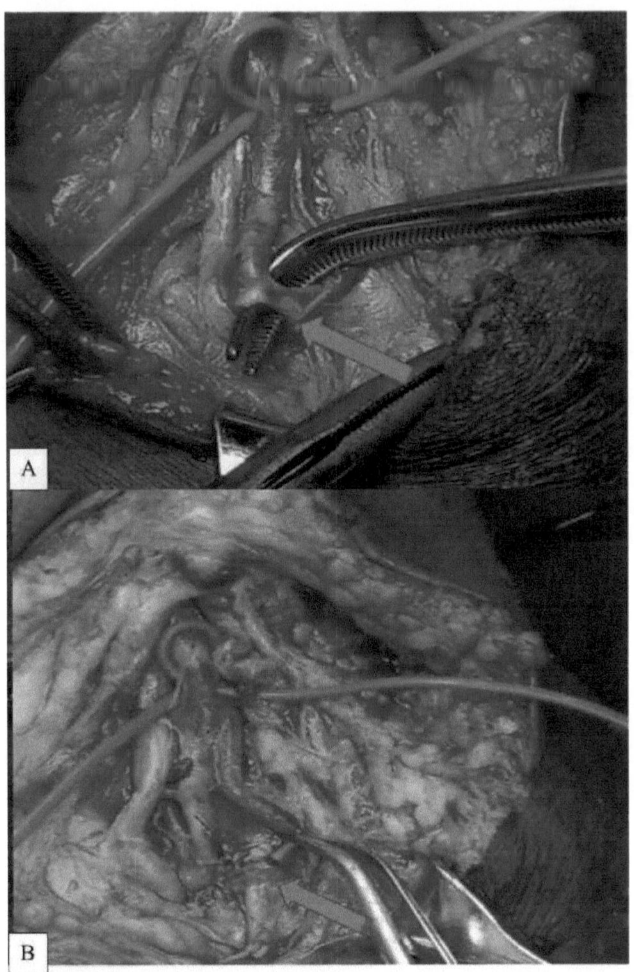

Figure 25: Photographs of the surgery, showing a connection between the right brachial artery and basilic vein (A) and overpressure of the arteriovenous shunt with 6/0 prolene (B).

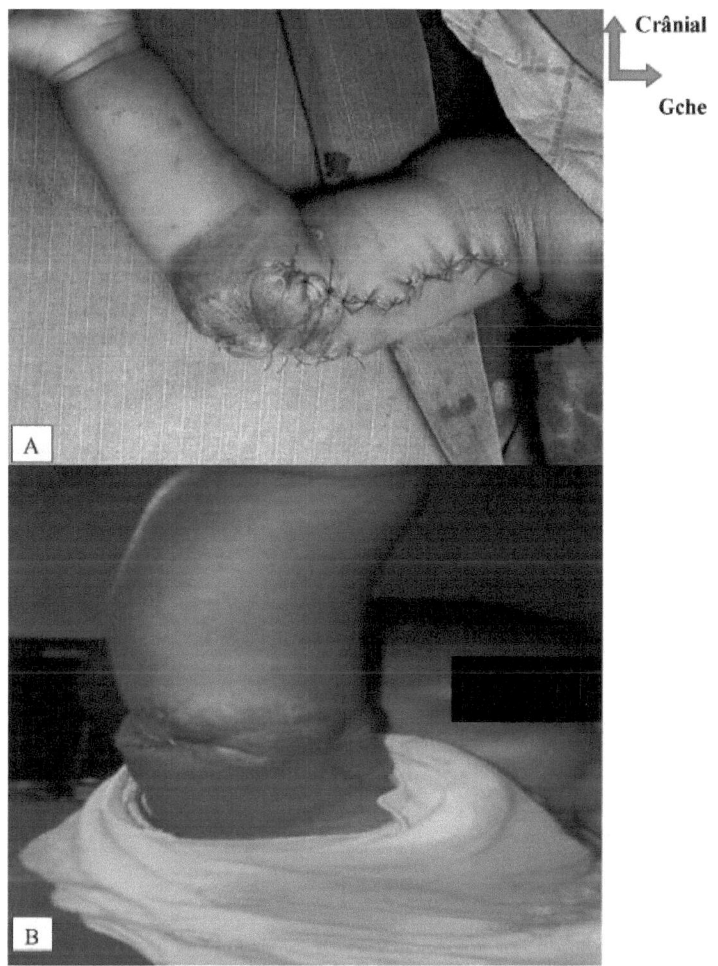

Figure 26: Immediate (A) and remote (B) post-operative photos of the right elbow.

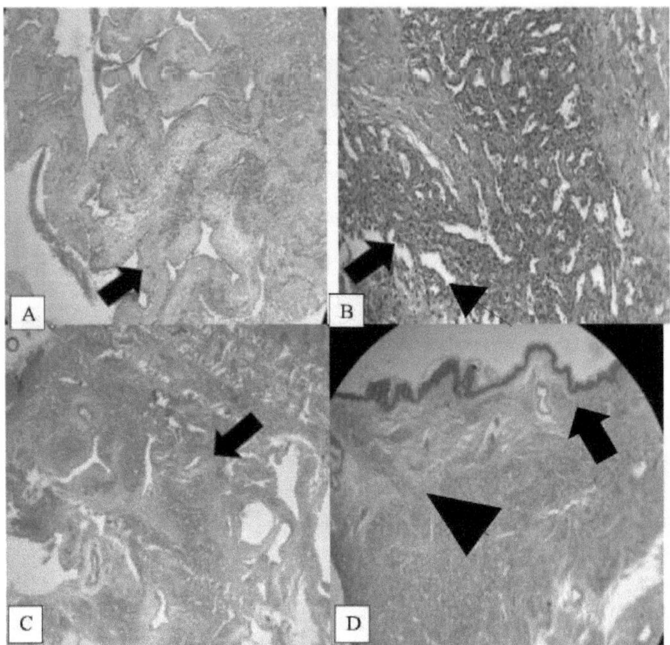

Figure 27: Histology of the surgical specimen confirming the AVM

A: Arterial dilatation with wall thickening.
B: Multiplication of venules (arrow) and cell without atypia (arrowhead).
C: Connections between arteries and veins.
D: Fibrous connective tissue (arrow) and regular skin tissue (arrowhead)

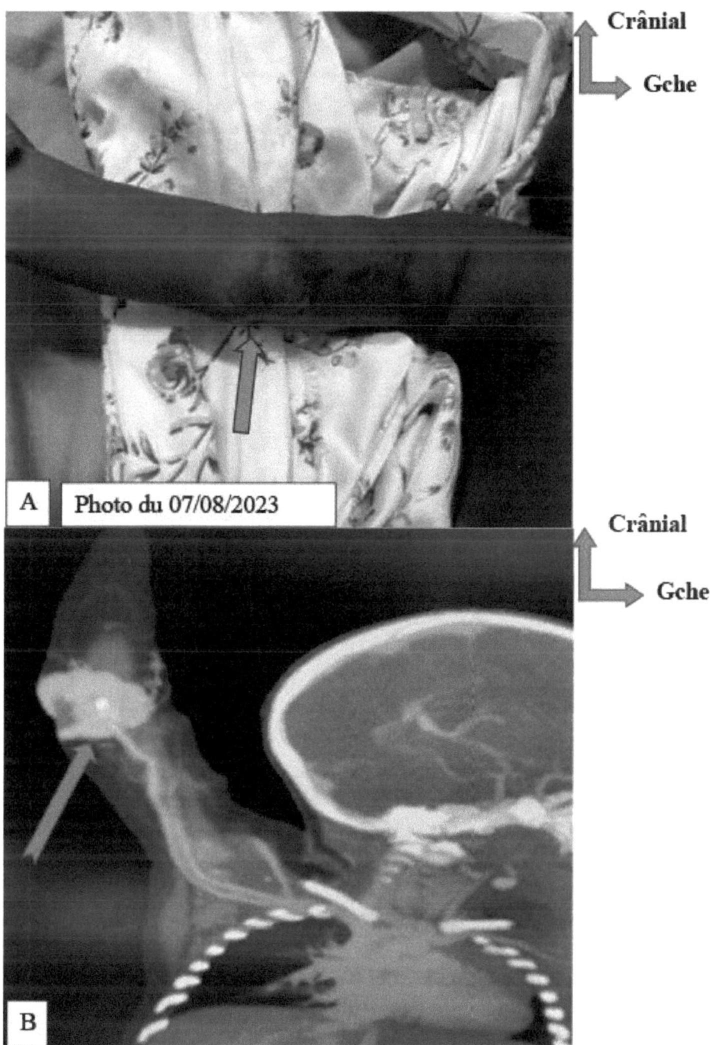

Figure 28: Control images after 07 months of surgery showing erythematous soft swelling of the right elbow (A) and persistence of the right elbow AVM after surgery (B).

CHAPTER 3

3. DISCUSSIONS

3.1.Limitations and difficulties :

During the course of this study, we encountered the following difficulties:

✓ The lack of an adequate technical platform for the management of vascular anomalies, in particular interventional radiology for embolisations.

✓ Breakdowns in the radiological equipment (scanner and lack of automatic injector) in our department. Because of this last difficulty, our study was delayed and we were obliged to take our patient to another facility to perform the control scan. It should be noted that all these angioscans were performed without an automatic injector, i.e. using a manual injection.

3.2.Frequency :

Arteriovenous malformation results from embryonic vasculogenesis and defective angiogenesis, leading to abnormal communication between arteries and veins that bypass the high-resistance capillary bed [8].

AVMs are a rare form of vascular malformation and their extra-cerebral and extra-spinal locations are rare (5-10%) [2].

3.3.Age of discovery :

AVMs develop during foetal life, but only 40-60% of them will be recognised at birth, and 30% will become apparent during childhood, peaking at puberty [10].

AVMs are congenital lesions that grow with the child and never disappear spontaneously, even in adulthood [10].

The majority of cases are diagnosed before the age of 30 [9].

In our study, the malformation was discovered at birth.

In Madagascar, F. Raherinantenaina reported a case of stage II arteriovenous malformation of the elbow in a 27-year-old woman in 2010 [8].

In France, Michel Wassef [27] found a case of arteriovenous malformation of the lower left lip in a 29-year-old woman in 2011, confirmed by histology.

Burrows et al [33] reported a case of pharmacological treatment of diffuse arteriovenous malformations of the right upper limb and shoulder in an infant aged 08 months.

In 2018, in Morocco, M. Bouayad et al [34] reported a case of association of superficial arteriovenous malformation, bi-condylar exostosis and a calcified synovial cyst of the elbow, in a 20-year-old young man.

3.4.Gender :

Arteriovenous malformations affect all areas of the skin, without gender predominance. Our case involved a female.

3.5.Family history :

We found no family history in our case. Of all vascular malformations, they are the most unpredictable and the most dangerous. Fortunately, they are rare and generally considered to be sporadic [3]. However, a few familial cases have been reported [12].

The genetic pathogenesis underlying the development of this malformation is currently accepted by some authors. A mutation in the *RASA-1* gene has been found in families of patients with a combination of multiple capillary malformations and arteriovenous fistulae or malformations, or Parkes Weber syndromes [12,13].

The literature reports cases of pulmonary AVMs in hereditary haemorrhagic telangiectasia (HHT), or Rendu-Osler Weber disease, affecting approximately 10 to 20 individuals in 100,000. It is an autosomal dominant disease, characterised by the presence of multiple cutaneous, mucosal and/or visceral arteriovenous malformations. Pulmonary arteriovenous malformations (PAVMs) carry a risk of rupture, a source of haemoptysis or haemothorax which can be fatal, with a complication rate of 50% according to LACOMBE et al [35].

Peutz-Jeghers syndrome (PJS) is rarer, with a prevalence of between 1 in 25,000 and 1 in 280,000. It is an autosomal dominant inherited disorder characterised by digestive hamartomatous polyps, mucocutaneous melanin pigmentation and a high risk of cancer. Most AVMs are hereditary, with a rate of between 80% and 95% in patients with hereditary haemorrhagic telangiectasia (HHT). Priscila Jijón et al reported a case of pulmonary arteriovenous malformation and Peutz-Jeghers syndrome in a 09-year-old girl. [36].

A case of capillary malformation, arteriovenous malformation type 2, was diagnosed in a 09-year-old boy who presented with multiple telangiectasias that had appeared progressively since birth, both on the face and on the back of the hands. On the basis of this clinical presentation, a diagnosis of capillary malformation-arteriovenous malformation syndrome (MC-MAV) was suggested. Cerebral MRI angiography was performed and found to be normal. Genetic testing identified a heterozygous c.2512C>T, p. (Arg838Trp) missense substitution in exon 15 of the EPHB4 gene, confirming the diagnosis of MC-MAV type 2. MC-MAV syndrome is characterised by the presence of multiple cutaneous capillary malformations and, in some cases, associated arteriovenous malformations.

MC-MAV type 2 syndrome is inherited as an autosomal dominant disorder and is caused by loss-of-function mutations in EPHB4, whereas MC-MAV type 1 syndrome is caused by heterozygous loss-of-function mutations in RASA1 [37].

3.6.Clinical signs :

At the beginning of their evolution, AVMs may present as an elementary

cutaneous lesion with low or even normal flow [4].
Progression to the active phase is secondary to triggering factors such as infection, trauma and hormonal changes [4] during pregnancy [10].
At the end of their evolution, the formation of multiple arteriovenous microfistulas or nidus can lead to cardiac decompensation [12].
The natural history of these lesions goes through several stages, which were codified by Schöbinger in 1994 [8].
The first is a dormant stage in which the lesion is inconspicuous and stable. It may appear as tissue thickening or as a pink or red macule simulating a capillary malformation (false "plane angioma"). At this stage, an increase in local temperature, a flutter or thrill may sometimes be seen, as well as echodoppler abnormalities. Stage II, as seen here, is characterised by an increase in volume and apparent extension to previously "healthy" tissue. An increase in local temperature, beating, thrill and murmur are easily detected [11].
Stage III corresponds to the complications phase, with skin atrophy and ulceration due to the diversion of blood flow or vascular theft, pain and bleeding, which can sometimes be fatal. Stage IV corresponds to rare large lesions whose shunt effect leads to heart failure.
The diagnosis of AVMs is primarily clinical.

Table 3: Clinical classification of AVMs proposed by Schöbinger in 1994.

Stadium	**Description of the different development phases**
I	Quiescent phase: warm, pink or bluish spot with arteriovenous shunt confirmed by echodoppler.
II	Expansion phase: the lesion increases in size and becomes pulsatile, with a thrill and a tense, tortuous venous network.
III	Destruction phase: stage II complicated by skin lesions with necrosis, infection, haemorrhage and pain
IV	Decompensation phase: stage III with heart failure

Clinically, we found a soft bluish non-ulcerating mass in the elbow with thrill on palpation but no pain. This is different from that reported by Tarik Abaaziz et al at the Hassan II University Hospital in Fez [33], who had identified a case of giant femoral arteriovenous malformation evolving since birth, characterised by a progressive increase in size and pain in the mass [33].

3.7.Imaging :

An echodoppler is essential to confirm the diagnosis by demonstrating a rapid-flow arteriovenous shunt.
The lesion consists of a "nidus" of abnormal vessels fed and drained by one or more arteries and veins dilated by the increased flow. This nidus allows arterial

and venous vessels to communicate with each other, with "early venous return" on arteriography [11].

MRI with vascular sequences can be used to determine the extension and development of the feeder vessels [38,39]. In the absence of specialised imaging, AVMs may be diagnosed clinically as hypervascular tumours, angiomas or venous malformations [11].

In principle, AVMs must be differentiated from simple arteriovenous fistulas, in which an artery and a vein communicate without the interposition of a nidus. It has a very different course. If there is any doubt, the clinical course of the malformation will provide diagnostic certainty [11].

In our case, we performed an echodoppler and then a CT angio of the upper limbs, which gave satisfactory results. Although MRI is the reference examination for diagnosis, we would also say that angiography-CT remains an effective alternative in the absence of MRI.

This result is consistent with the literature, in the study by Tarik Abaaziz et al at the Hassan II University Hospital in Fez [40]. A case of giant femoral arteriovenous malformation was reported in a 20-year-old patient. An angioscan showed an arteriovenous malformation (AVM) with early venous return. Arteriography revealed a left scarpal AVM supplied by branches of the deep femoral artery, branches of the superficial femoral artery, branches of the homolateral hypogastric artery and branches of the common femoral artery. Embolisation was performed by retrograde puncture of the contralateral common femoral artery, with a significant reduction in the volume of the malformation [40].

In France, Humeau-Heurtier et al [41] reported in 2017, for the first time, the use of ILS for the reproducible exploration of an AVM of the left upper limb in a 07-month-old infant.

ILS is a non-invasive microvascular imaging technology that enables precise mapping of vascular lesions such as incipient AVMs at the stage when they may clinically appear to be flat angiomas. It is easy to use and the absence of direct contact with the skin means that microvascular flows can be respected. This examination, which is perfectly reproducible, makes it possible to initiate imaging follow-up in parallel with the clinic and to space out MRI scans with GA [41].

3.8.Treatment

In the case of a confirmed AVM, the therapeutic approach depends on the clinical stage of the disease at the time of discovery, and must be adapted throughout the course of the disease [18].

Classically, small, quiescent AVMs (Schöbinger stage I) should not be operated

on or resected carcinologically [8].
Surgery is mainly reserved for progressive or complicated forms (stages II to IV). This surgical procedure must allow complete eradication of the lesion. Otherwise, incomplete excision may lead to recurrence, or even worsening of the disease, sometimes with life-threatening consequences [8].
Complete removal of the lesion by embolisation and/or surgery is often not feasible, and incomplete resection can lead to worsening of the AVMs [6]. As they develop, these vascular malformations infiltrate the surrounding tissues, considerably impairing patients' quality of life and, in the most serious cases, threatening their prognosis. Arteriovenous malformations pose a diagnostic problem. This is probably due to the nosological problem associated with vascular malformations [8].
In our case, we performed open surgery, which was successful, but a check-up after 07 months showed reconstitution of the arteriovenous malformation with no other signs of associated complications.
Janot et al, followed 125 peripheral superficial AVMs, of which 68 patients had been embolised at least once and 26 patients with facial AVMs had been treated endovascularly. The clinical presentation was marked by significant lesion polymorphism. The management of these patients must take into account the mucocutaneous involvement of the lesion, and the potential functional and aesthetic damage. Vital prognosis may also be at risk in the event of haemorrhagic complications. A complete cure is sometimes possible, whereas in other cases treatment will be symptomatic only [42].
Gregor M. Dunham et al in 2016 in Washington [32], found two cases of grade III superficial arteriovenous Schobinger malformations, one in a 58-year-old woman with a uterine AVM and the other in a 45-year-old woman with an AVM of the elbow, which were treated by embolisation.
A study analysing 341 articles including the term 'haemangioma' in the title or abstract, and published in PubMed in 2009, concluded that the term was incorrectly used in 71.3% of publications. And patients whose lesions were mislabelled were obviously more likely to receive inappropriate treatment (20.6%), compared with those whose lesions were correctly diagnosed using ISSVA terminology (0.0%; $P < 0.001$). This misuse of the term "haemangioma" was independent of discipline and author, with errors occurring in paediatrics (60.0%), internal medicine (61.4%), emergency (68.9%) and obstetrics and gynaecology (70%) ($P = 0.68$) [30].

3.9.Histology

Histologically, an AVM consists of arteries and veins of recognisable structure, generally with a media thickness proportionate to their lumen. These various

vessels, generally round or oval in shape, are dispersed fairly evenly throughout the host tissue, often associated with fibrosis simulating a vascular tumour [11].
The dermis and underlying soft tissues are occupied by a large number of medium-sized vessels, usually regularly rounded, of intermediate structure, with no individualisable elastic framework. This large component of medium-sized vessels is associated with capillary proliferation, which is more marked between the muscle bundles of the orbicularis and in certain areas of the dermis. This capillary component is discretely lobulated in places, but more often forms irregularly contoured clusters. There is significant collagen sclerosis, particularly deep down and laterally. Elsewhere, especially in the muscle, there is discrete lipomatosis. A few spherical emboli are found [27].
We performed histology on the surgical specimen, which revealed vascular dilatation with fibrosis of the surrounding connective tissue, with no sign of malignancy. This is in line with the literature.

CHAPTER 4

CONCLUSION

Superficial vascular malformations are relatively rare and often unrecognised. Their classification is essential to avoid diagnostic and therapeutic errors.

Angiography-CT is an effective approach, although it can cause radiation. Doppler ultrasound and MRI angiography are ideal for diagnosis. Management is multidisciplinary.

RECOMMENDATIONS

We recommend that the administrative authorities provide medical imaging departments with the necessary materials for interventional radiology and ensure regular maintenance of radiology equipment.

REFERENCES

1. Barreau G., Marmat F., Gariel V. et al, Intracranial AVM, Radio Journal, Diagnosis and Intervention, 95.12 (2014): 1161-1174.

2. Dahhouki S. Les malformations vasculaires : Étude prospective au sein du service de dermatologie de CHU de Fès ; Mem. Maroc (2020) :333.

3. Cappabianca S, Del Vecchio W, Giudice A and coll. vascular malformations of the tongue: MRI findings on three cases. Dentomaxillofac Radiol (2006), 35: 205-208.

4. Vanwijcka R, Dégardin-Capon N. Arteriovenous malformations: clinical aspects and evolution. Ann Chir Plast Esthet (2006) ; 51 :440-6.

5. Massager N., Lonneville S., Mine B. et al. Results of Gamma Knife radiosurgical treatment of cerebral arteriovenous malformations, Rev Med Brux. (2016), 37 : 18-25.

6. Gelbert F., Merland J., Vargas M. et al. Medullary vascular malformations, Imaging the spine and spinal cord. Masson (2017); 9: 99.

7. Bataille, A. C., and Boon, L. M.,Clinical aspects of capillary malformations, Ann Chir.Plast Esthet, (2006), 51(4-5): 347-56.

8. Raherinantenaina F., Rajaonanahary T.M.A., Rakotomena S.D. et al. Schöbinger stage II arteriovenous malformation of the left upper limb: a case report from Madagascar. Annales de Cardiologie et d'Angéiologie. Edition Masson, (2013) :183.

9. Söderman M, Andersson T, Karlsson B and al. Management of patients with brain arteriovenous malformations. Eur Journal Radiol (2003); 46: 195-205

10. Odile Enjolras, Véronique Soupre. Classification of superficial vascular anomalies. Arnold-Netter, 75012 Paris, France. Elsevier Masson SAS. Presse Med (2010); 39: 457-464.

1. Brevière G ; Degrugillier-Chopinet C ; Bisdorff-Bresson A., Superficial vascular anomalies. EMC - Cardiologie (2011), 6(1) : 1-21.

12. Das, Abanti, et al. Vascular anomalies: nomenclature, classification and imaging algorithms." Acta Radiologica 64.2 (2023): 837-849.

13. Deklunder G., Dauzat M., Boivin V. et al, Exploration des vaisseaux du membre supérieur. Doppler et échotomographie. EMC-Radiologie, 1.6 (2004): 632-646.

14. Moure C, Reynaert G, Lehmman P et al. Classification of superficial vascular tumours: basis of the classification and clinical interest. Masson, Rev. Stomatol Chir Maxillofac (2007); 108:201-209.

15. OUSI B. Journées Parisiennes du groupe laser de la société française de dermatologie. Paris 1-2June 2007: Treatment of adult flat angiomas by laser KTP (2007); 26 (16): 34-38.

16. Organ of the French dermatology society and the association of French-speaking dermatologists. Angioma. Annale de Dermatologie et de vénérologie (2005) ; 132 (10) :172-176
17. Enjolras, O. "Superficial vascular anomalies: the "angiomas". Encycl Med Chir. (2001) : 98-745.
18. Casanova D, Bardot J, Bartoli J-M et al. Surgical treatment of arteriovenous malformations. Ann Chir. Plast. Esthet (2006) ; 51 :456- 70.
19. Dubois J, Soulez G, Oliva VL, Berthiaume MJ, Lapierre C, Therasse E. Soft-tissue venous malformations in adult patients: imaging and therapeutic issues. Radiographics 21.6 (2001): 1519-1531.
20. Koeller KK, Alamo L, Adair CF, Smirniotopoulos JG. Congenital cystic masses of the neck: radiologic-pathologic correlation. Radiographics (1999); 19:121-46.
21. Enjolras, O. "What's new in angiomas? Infantile vascular tumours1." Les Nouvelles dermatologiques 22.9 (2003): 602-604.
22. Trop I, Dubois J, Guibaud L, et al. Soft-tissue venous malformations in pediatric and young adult patients: diagnosis with Doppler US. Radiology 212.3 (1999): 841-845.
23. T. MOSER, R. CHAPOT, C. JAHN et al. Imagerie des anomalies vasculaires des tissus mous : diagnostic et traitement, Masson, Paris, Feuillets de Radiologie 45.1 (2005) : 13-36.
24. Enjolras O. Angiomas and angiomatoses. Presse Med (2010) ; 39 :454-6
25. M. Barreau, A. Dompmartin. Non-syndromic vascular skin malformations. Annals of dermatology and venereology (2014) 141, 5667.
26. Michael Naouri, Gérard Lorettea, Charlotte Barbier et al. Malformations artérioveineuses, mise au point ; Masson SAS Presse Med (2010) ; 39 : 465-470.
27. Michel wassef. A case of arteriovenous malformation of the lip. Elsevier Masson, Annales de pathologie (2011) 31, 292-296.
28. Theiler M, Walchli R, WeibelL: Vascular anomalies-a practical approach. JDDG (2013); 11: 397-405.
29. Seront E, Valérie D., Julien C. et al. Vascular malformations: new hope thanks to anti-tumour targeted therapies. Louvain médical (2022), 141 : 261.
30. Hassanein A, Mulliken JB, Fishman S, Greene AK: Evaluation of Terminology for Vascular Anomalies in Current Literature. PlastReconstrSurg (2011) ; 127 : 347-51.
31. Sara M.B, Helia R, Giorgio L et al. Arteriovenous malformations: complex management. Rev Med Suisse (2018); 14: 2214-9.
32. Dunham G., Christopher R., Vaidya S., Finding the Nidus: Detection and Workup of Non-Central Nervous System Arteriovenous Malformations,

Radiographics (2016); 36: 891-903.

33. Patricia E., Burrows John B., Mulliken, Steven J. et al, pharmacological treatment of a diffuse arteriovenous malformation of the upper extremity in a child, The Journal of Craniofacial Surgery & Volume 20, Supplement 1 (2009): 567-602.

34. M. Bouayad, B. Lekehal, S. El Khaloufia et al. Arteriovenous malformation, a bi-condylar exostosis and calcified synovial cyst of the elbow: Association or coincidence? Masson Journal de Traumatologie du Sport 28 (2011) : 247-250.

35. Lacombe P., Lacout A., Marcy P.Y. et al. Diagnosis and treatment of pulmonary arteriovenous malformations in hereditary haemorrhagic telangiectasia: a general review. Journal of Diagnostic and Interventional Radiology (2013), 94: 847-861.

36. Jij0n, P., Marolleau, F., Shango-Lody La Ndjeka Pasu, P. et al. Pulmonary arteriovenous malformation and Peutz-Jeghers syndrome: review of the literature and discussion of development, follow-up and treatment. Medical Leuven (2018), 137: 370.

37. Cheumaga, Franck Aurelien Chouamou, et al. "Occipital arteriovenous malformation: about a case report." PAMJ-Clinical Medicine 4.5 (2020): 2-3.

38. Mulliken JB, Glowaki J. Hemangiomas and vascular malformations in infants and children: A classification based on endothelial characteristics. Plast Reconstruction Surg (1982); 62: 412-22.

39. Barsky SH, Rosen S, Geer DE, Noe JM. The nature and evolution of port wine stains: a computer-assisted study. J Invest Dermatol (1980) ,74 :154- 7.

40. Abaaziz, T, Jiber H, Bouarhroum, Abdellatif. Giant femoral arteriovenous malformation. Blood Thrombosis Vessels (2018), 30: 43-44.

41. Humeau Heurtier Λ, Martin l, Bazeries P, et al. Speckle laser imaging of an arteriovenous malformation in an infant. In: Annals of Dermatology and Venereology. Elsevier Masson (2017): 174-175.

42. Janot K., Herbreteau D., Maruani A. et al. Periorbital arteriovenous malformations: dangerousness and management. Journal of Neuroradiology (2018), 45: 95-96.

Summary

Arteriovenous malformations (AVMs) are fast-flowing vascular lesions resulting from abnormal communication between the arterial and venous systems without vascularisation of the normal capillary network. Peripheral locations are rare (5-10%) and are recognised at birth (40-60%).

Objective:

To determine the contribution of angio-CT in the diagnosis of arteriovenous malformation in newborns.

Observation :

The baby was female, 15 days old, the result of a normal full-term pregnancy and an eutoctopic vaginal delivery. There were no other associated anomalies and no particular family history.

At birth, he presented with a raised, regular, bluish, erythematous skin mass on the posteromedial aspect of the right elbow, with pulsatile thrills on palpation. An initial echodoppler diagnosed an AVM. Arterial and venous angio-CT with IV of 10ml omnipaque 350mg was performed. It showed vascular dilatation with subcutaneous arteriovenous communication on the posteromedial aspect of the right elbow, creating a mass (nidus) measuring 61x46mm. This mass was supplied by the right brachial artery with an arteriovenous fistula between the latter and the homolateral basilic vein upstream of the mass. It was drained by the homolateral basilic vein. The cephalic vein was slightly dilated with no arteriovenous fistula. There were small arterial branches emanating from the brachial artery in the forearm. The vascular lesions were confirmed intraoperatively. There were no immediate postoperative complications. A check-up after 07 months revealed a recurrence of the AVM.

Conclusion:

Peripheral arteriovenous malformations are rare in neonates. Angio-CT is an effective approach, although it can cause radiation. Doppler ultrasound and MRI are the ideal diagnostic tests.

KEYWORDS: Angioscan, AVM of the elbow, Newborn, Mali Hospital

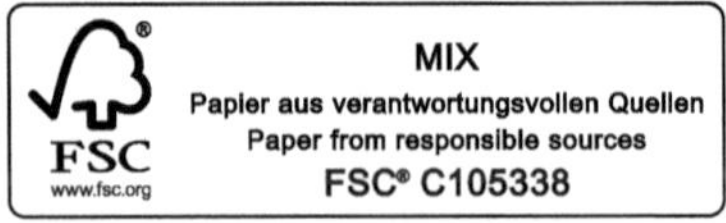

Printed by Books on Demand GmbH, Norderstedt / Germany